Christopher B. Keys
Peter W. Dowrick
Editors

People with Disabilities: Empowerment and Community Action

People with Disabilities: Empowerment and Community Action has been co-published simultaneously as *Journal of Prevention & Intervention in the Community* Volume 21, Number 2 2001.

Pre-publication
REVIEWS,
COMMENTARIES,
EVALUATIONS . . .

"**L**ooks at three mutually exclusive constructs for fostering community action to meet the needs of a wide range of individuals with disabilities to achieve meaningful membership and partcipation in their communities."

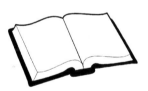

Preston Lewis, MA
Program Manager
Division of Exceptional
Children Services
Kentucky Department
of Education

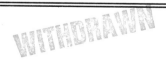

More pre-publication
REVIEWS, COMMENTARIES, EVALUATIONS . . .

"Timely and useful . . . provides valuable lessons and guidance for everyone involved in the disability movement. This book is a must read for researchers and practitioners interested in disability rights issues!"

Karen M. Ward, EdD
Director
Center for Human Development
Associate Professor
University of Alaska, Anchorage

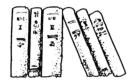

"Groundbreaking . . . uses state-of-the-art community approaches to promote both scientific research and social justice for people with disabilities. A variety of innovative strategies . . . excellent . . . should be required reading for anyone interested in disabilities issues and community research."

Stephanie Riger, PhD
Professor of Psychology,
Gender, and Women's Studies
University of Illinois at Chicago

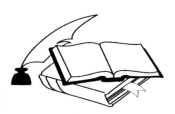

More pre-publication
REVIEWS, COMMENTARIES, EVALUATIONS . . .

"There is much rhetoric these days about university-community partnerships, empowerment, and participatory action research. This book shows how to translate these lofty ideals into practice. It does so by presenting a variety of intervention models and then showing how each was implemented in actual community settings. There are contributions from many of the leading scholars in the field–a veritable 'who's who' of community psychologists interested in disabilities."

Cary Cherniss, PhD
Professor of Applied Psychology
Rutgers University
President, Society
for Community Research
and Action (Division 27
of the American Psychological
Association)

"Offers practical insight on how to: gain entry and acceptance within the community; facilitate discussions to identify areas of need; develop, promote, and implement effective programs; and evaluate the effects of programs. Whether you're a community psychologist or a professional interested in effective pertnerships targeting important issues, this book will have useful information for you!"

Martin J. Ikeda, PhD
Coordinator of Research
& Special Projects
Heartland AEA 11
Johnston, Iowa

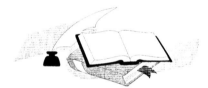

More pre-publication
REVIEWS, COMMENTARIES, EVALUATIONS . . .

"**O**ffers models and examples of how people with disabilities can participate in and influence the work of understanding and influencing conditions affecting independent living. In de-mystifying action research in the field of disability, this text helps us see our common works of building communities worthy of all of us."

Stephen B. Fawcett, PhD
University Distinguished Professor
of Human Development
University of Texas

The Haworth Press, Inc.

People with Disabilities: Empowerment and Community Action

People with Disabilities: Empowerment and Community Action has been co-published simultaneously as *Journal of Prevention & Intervention in the Community*™, Volume 21, Number 2 2001.

The *Journal of Prevention & Intervention in the Community*™ Monographic "Separates" (formerly the Prevention in Human Services series)*

For information on previous issues of Prevention in Human Services, edited by Robert E. Hess, please contact: The Haworth Press, Inc., 10 Alice Street, Binghamton, NY 13904-1580 USA.

Below is a list of "separates," which in serials librarianship means a special issue simultaneously published as a special journal issue or double-issue *and* as a "separate" hardbound monograph. (This is a format which we also call a "DocuSerial.")

"Separates" are published because specialized libraries or professionals may wish to purchase a specific thematic issue by itself in a format which can be separately cataloged and shelved, as opposed to purchasing the journal on an on-going basis. Faculty members may also more easily consider a "separate" for classroom adoption.

"Separates" are carefully classified separately with the major book jobbers so that the journal tie-in can be noted on new book order slips to avoid duplicate purchasing.

You may wish to visit Haworth's website at . . .

http://www.HaworthPress.com

. . . to search our online catalog for complete tables of contents of these separates and related publications.

You may also call 1-800-HAWORTH (outside US/Canada: 607-722-5857), or Fax 1-800-895-0582 (outside US/Canada: 607-771-0012), or e-mail at:

getinfo@haworthpressinc.com

People with Disabilities: Empowerment and Community Action, edited by Christopher B. Keys, PhD, and Peter W. Dowrick, PhD (Vol. 21(2), 2001).

Family Systems/Family Therapy: Applications for Clinical Practice, edited by Joan D. Atwood, PhD (Vol. 21, No. 1, 2001).

Diverse Families, Competent Families: Innovations in Research and Preventive Intervention Practice, edited by Janet F. Gillespie, PhD, and Judy Primavera, PhD (Vol. 20, No. 1/2, 2000). *Provides a portrait of the real lives and practical challenges of our nation's families as they face a new millenium. You will discover family adaptation and competence in a variety of contexts and situations such as day-to-day issues of coping and survival, as well as major milestones such as sending children off to school, becoming a caregiver for a family member, and more.*

Employment in Community Psychology: The Diversity of Opportunity, edited by Joseph R. Ferrari, PhD, and Clifford R. O'Donnel, PhD (Vol. 19, No. 2, 2000). *"Fascinating and instructive reading, indeed a must read for all community psychology faculty, students, and potential employers. Sixteen community psychologists offer compelling, diverse and unique perspectives on their employment journeys." (Kenneth I. Maton, PhD, Professor of Psychology, University of Maryland)*

HIV/AIDS Prevention: Current Issues in Community Practice, edited by Doreen D. Salina, PhD (Vol. 19, No. 1, 2000). *Helps researchers and psychologists explore specific methods of improving HIV/AIDS prevention research.*

Educating Students to Make-a-Difference: Community-Based Service Learning, edited by Joseph R. Ferrari, PhD, and Judith G. Chapman, PhD (Vol. 18(1/2), 1999). *"There is something here for everyone interested in the social psychology of service-learning." (Frank Bernt, PhD, Associate Professor, St. Joseph's University)*

Program Implementation in Preventive Trials, edited by Joseph A. Durlak and Joseph R. Ferrari, PhD (Vol. 17(2), 1998). *"Fills an important gap in preventive research. . . . Highlights an array of important questions related to implementation and demonstrates just how good community-based intervention programs can be when issues related to implementation are taken seriously." (Judy Primavera, PhD, Associate Professor of Psychology, Fairfield University, Fairfield, Connecticut)*

Preventing Drunk Driving, edited by Elsie R. Shore, PhD, and Joseph R. Ferrari, PhD (Vol. 17(1), 1998). *"A must read for anyone interested in reducing the needless injuries and death caused by the drunk driver."* (Terrance D. Schiavone, President, National Commission Against Drunk Driving, Washington, DC)

Manhood Development in Urban African-American Communities, edited by Roderick J. Watts, PhD, and Robert J. Jagers (Vol. 16(1/2), 1998). *"Watts and Jagers provide the much-needed foundational and baseline information and research that begins to philosophically and empirically validate the importance of understanding culture, oppression, and gender when working with males in urban African-American communities."* (Paul Hill, Jr., MSW, LISW, ACSW, East End Neighborhood House, Cleveland, Ohio)

Diversity Within the Homeless Population: Implications for Intervention, edited by Elizabeth M. Smith, PhD, and Joseph R. Ferrari, PhD (Vol. 15(2), 1997). *"Examines why homelessness is increasing, as well as treatment options, case management techniques, and community intervention programs that can be used to prevent homelessness."* (American Public Welfare Association)

Education in Community Psychology: Models for Graduate and Undergraduate Programs, edited by Clifford R. O'Donnell, PhD, and Joseph R. Ferrari, PhD (Vol. 15(1), 1997). *"An invaluable resource for students seeking graduate training in community psychology . . . [and will] also serve faculty who want to improve undergraduate teaching and graduate programs."* (Marybeth Shinn, PhD, Professor of Psychology and Coordinator, Community Doctoral Program, New York University, New York, New York)

Adolescent Health Care: Program Designs and Services, edited by John S. Wodarski, PhD, Marvin D. Feit, PhD, and Joseph R. Ferrari, PhD (Vol. 14(1/2), 1997). *Devoted to helping practitioners address the problems of our adolescents through the use of preventive interventions based on sound empirical data.*

Preventing Illness Among People with Coronary Heart Disease, edited by John D. Piette, PhD, Robert M. Kaplan, PhD, and Joseph R. Ferrari, PhD (Vol. 13(1/2), 1996). *"A useful contribution to the interaction of physical health, mental health, and the behavioral interventions for patients with CHD. "* (Public Health: The Journal of the Society of Public Health)

Sexual Assault and Abuse: Sociocultural Context of Prevention, edited by Carolyn F. Swift, PhD* (Vol. 12(2), 1995). *"Delivers a cornucopia for all who are concerned with the primary prevention of these damaging and degrading acts."* (George J. McCall, PhD, Professor of Sociology and Public Administration, University of Missouri)

International Approaches to Prevention in Mental Health and Human Services, edited by Robert E. Hess, PhD, and Wolfgang Stark* (Vol. 12(1), 1995.) *Increases knowledge of prevention strategies from around the world.*

Self-Help and Mutual Aid Groups: International and Multicultural Perspectives, edited by Francine Lavoie, PhD, Thomasina Borkman, PhD, and Benjamin Gidron* (Vol. 11(1/2), 1995). *"A helpful orientation and overview, as well as useful data and methodological suggestions."* (International Journal of Group Psychotherapy)

Prevention and School Transitions, edited by Leonard A. Jason, PhD, Karen E. Danner, and Karen S. Kurasaki, MA* (Vol. 10(2), 1994). *"A collection of studies by leading ecological and systems-oriented theorists in the area of school transitions, describing the stressors, personal resources available, and coping strategies among different groups of children and adolescents undergoing school transitions."* (Reference & Research Book News)

Religion and Prevention in Mental Health: Research, Vision, and Action, edited by Kenneth I. Pargament, PhD, Kenneth I. Maton, PhD, and Robert E. Hess, PhD* (Vol. 9(2) & 10(1), 1992). *"The authors provide an admirable framework for considering the important, yet often overlooked, differences in theological perspectives."* (Family Relations)

Families as Nurturing Systems: Support Across the Life Span, edited by Donald G. Unger, PhD, and Douglas R. Powell, PhD* (Vol. 9(1), 1991). *"A useful book for anyone thinking about alternative ways of delivering a mental health service."* (British Journal of Psychiatry)

Ethical Implications of Primary Prevention, edited by Gloria B. Levin, PhD, and Edison J. Trickett, PhD (Vol. 8(2), 1991). *"A thoughtful and thought-provoking summary of ethical issues related to intervention programs and community research."* (Betty Tableman, MPA, Director, Division of Prevention Services and Demonstration Projects, Michigan Department of Mental Health, Lansing) Here is the first systematic and focused treatment of the ethical implications of primary prevention practice and research.

Career Stress in Changing Times, edited by James Campbell Quick, PhD, MBA, Robert E. Hess, PhD, Jared Hermalin, PhD, and Jonathan D. Quick, MD* (Vol. 8(1), 1990). *"A well-organized book. . . . It deals with planning a career and career changes and the stresses involved. " (American Association of Psychiatric Administrators)*

Prevention in Community Mental Health Centers, edited by Robert E. Hess, PhD, and John Morgan, PhD* (Vol. 7(2), 1990). *"A fascinating bird's-eye view of six significant programs of preventive care which have survived the rise and fall of preventive psychiatry in the U.S." (British Journal of Psychiatry)*

Protecting the Children: Strategies for Optimizing Emotional and Behavioral Development, edited by Raymond P. Lorion, PhD* (Vol. 7(1), 1990). *"This is a masterfully conceptualized and edited volume presenting theory-driven, empirically based, developmentally oriented prevention. " (Michael C. Roberts, PhD, Professor of Psychology, The University of Alabama)*

The National Mental Health Association: Eighty Years of Involvement in the Field of Prevention, edited by Robert E. Hess, PhD, and Jean DeLeon, PhD* (Vol. 6(2), 1989). *"As a family life educator interested in both the history of the field, current efforts, and especially the evaluation of programs, I find this book quite interesting. I enjoyed reviewing it and believe that I will return to it many times. It is also a book I will recommend to students." (Family Relations)*

A Guide to Conducting Prevention Research in the Community: First Steps, James G. Kelly, PhD, Nancy Dassoff, PhD, Ira Levin, PhD, Janice Schreckengost, MA, AB, Stephen P. Stelzner, PhD, and B. Eileen Altman, PhD* (Vol. 6(1), 1989). *"An invaluable compendium for the prevention practitioner, as well as the researcher, laying out the essentials for developing effective prevention programs in the community. . . . . This is a book which should be in the prevention practitioner's library, to read, re-read, and ponder." (The Community Psychologist)*

Prevention: Toward a Multidisciplinary Approach, edited by Leonard A. Jason, PhD, Robert D. Felner, PhD, John N. Moritsugu, PhD, and Robert E. Hess, PhD* (Vol. 5(2), 1987). *"Will not only be of intellectual value to the professional but also to students in courses aimed at presenting a refreshingly comprehensive picture of the conceptual and practical relationships between community and prevention." (Seymour B. Sarason, Associate Professor of Psychology, Yale University)*

Prevention and Health: Directions for Policy and Practice, edited by Alfred H. Katz, PhD, Jared A. Hermalin, PhD, and Robert E. Hess, PhD* (Vol. 5(1), 1987). *Read about the most current efforts being undertaken to promote better health.*

The Ecology of Prevention: Illustrating Mental Health Consultation, edited by James G. Kelly, PhD, and Robert E. Hess, PhD* (Vol. 4(3/4), 1987). *"Will provide the consultant with a very useful framework and the student with an appreciation for the time and commitment necessary to bring about lasting changes of a preventive nature." (The Community Psychologist)*

Beyond the Individual: Environmental Approaches and Prevention, edited by Abraham Wandersman, PhD, and Robert E. Hess, PhD* (Vol. 4(1/2), 1985). *"This excellent book has immediate appeal for those involved with environmental psychology . . . likely to be of great interest to those working in the areas of community psychology, planning, and design." (Australian Journal of Psychology)*

Prevention: The Michigan Experience, edited by Betty Tableman, MPA, and Robert E. Hess, PhD* (Vol. 3(4), 1985). *An in-depth look at one state's outstanding prevention programs.*

Studies in Empowerment: Steps Toward Understanding and Action, edited by Julian Rappaport, Carolyn Swift, Robert E. Hess, PhD* (Vol. 3(2/3), 1984). *"Provides diverse applications of the empowerment model to the promotion of mental health and the prevention of mental illness." (Prevention Forum Newsline)*

Aging and Prevention: New Approaches for Preventing Health and Mental Health Problems in Older Adults, edited by Sharon P. Simson, Laura Wilson, Jared Hermalin, PhD, and Robert E. Hess, PhD (Vol. 3(1), 1983). *"Highly recommended for professionals and laymen interested in modern viewpoints and techniques for avoiding many physical and mental health problems of the elderly. Written by highly qualified contributors with extensive experience in their respective fields." (The Clinical Gerontologist)*

Strategies for Needs Assessment in Prevention, edited by Alex Zautra, Kenneth Bachrach, and Robert E. Hess, PhD* (Vol. 2(4), 1983). *"An excellent survey on applied techniques for doing needs assessments. . . It should be on the shelf of anyone involved in prevention." (Journal of Pediatric Psychology)*

Innovations in Prevention:, edited by Robert E. Hess, PhD, and Jared Hermalin, PhD* (Vol. 2(3), 1983). *An exciting book that provides invaluable insights on effective prevention programs.*

Rx Television: Enhancing the Preventive Impact of TV, edited by Joyce Sprafkin, Carolyn Swift, PhD, and Robert E. Hess, PhD* (Vol. 2(1/2), 1983). *"The successful interventions reported in this volume make interesting reading on two grounds. First, they show quite clearly how powerful television can be in molding children. Second, they illustrate how this power can be used for good ends." (Contemporary Psychology)*

Early Intervention Programs for Infants, edited by Howard A. Moss, MD, Robert E. Hess, PhD, and Carolyn Swift, PhD* (Vol. 1(4), 1982). *"A useful resource book for those child psychiatrists, paediatricians, and psychologists interested in early intervention and prevention." (The Royal College of Psychiatrists)*

Helping People to Help Themselves: Self-Help and Prevention, edited by Leonard D. Borman, PhD, Leslie E. Borck, PhD, Robert E. Hess, PhD, and Frank L. Pasquale* (Vol. 1(3), 1982). *"A timely volume . . . a mine of information for interested clinicians, and should stimulate those wishing to do systematic research in the self-help area." (The Journal of Nervous and Mental Disease)*

Evaluation and Prevention in Human Services, edited by Jared Hermalin, PhD, and Jonathan A. Morell, PhD* (Vol. 1(1/2), 1982). *Features methods and problems related to the evaluation of prevention programs.*

People with Disabilities: Empowerment and Community Action
has been co-published simultaneously as *Journal of Prevention &
Intervention in the Community*™, Volume 21, Number 2 2001.

Cover design by Thomas J. Mayshock Jr.

The Haworth Press, Inc., 10 Alice Street, Binghamton, NY 13904-1580 USA

Library of Congress Cataloging-in-Publication Data

People with disabilities: empowerment and community action / Christopher B. Keys, Peter W.
Dowrick, editors.
     p. cm.
     "Co-published simultaneously as Journal of prevention & intervention in the community,
volume 21, number 2 2001."
     Includes bibliographical references and index.
     ISBN 0-7890-1310-X (alk. paper)–ISBN 0-7890-1311-8 (alk. paper)
     1. Handicapped–Services for. 2. Community health services–Citizen participation. 3. Com-
munity organization. I. Keys, Christopher. II. Dowrick, Peter W. III. Journal of prevention & intervention in the community.

HV1568 .P445 2001
362.4′048–dc21
                                          2001016698

People with Disabilities: Empowerment and Community Action

Christopher B. Keys
Peter W. Dowrick
Editors

People with Disabilities: Empowerment and Community Action has been co-published simultaneously as *Journal of Prevention & Intervention in the Community*™, Volume 21, Number 2 2001.

The Haworth Press, Inc.
New York • London • Oxford

Indexing, Abstracting & Website/Internet Coverage

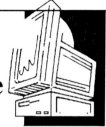

This section provides you with a list of major indexing & abstracting services. That is to say, each service began covering this periodical during the year noted in the right column. Most Websites which are listed below have indicated that they will either post, disseminate, compile, archive, cite or alert their own Website users with research-based content from this work. (This list is as current as the copyright date of this publication.)

Abstracting, Website/Indexing Coverage .... Year When Coverage Began

- *Behavioral Medicine Abstracts* 1996

- *BUBL Information Service. An Internet-based Information Service for the UK higher education community <URL:http://bubl.ac.uk/>* 1996

- *CNPIEC Reference Guide: Chinese National Directory of Foreign Periodicals* 1996

- *EMBASE/Excerpta Medica Secondary Publishing Division <URL: http://www.elsevicr.nl>* 1999

- *Family Studies Database (online and CD/ROM) <www.nisc.com>* 1996

- *FINDEX <www.publist.com>* 1999

- *Gay & Lesbian Abstracts* 2000

(continued)

- *HealthPromis* 1997

- *IBZ International Bibliography of Periodical Literature* .. 1996

- *MANTIS (Manual, Alternative and Natural Therapy) MANTIS is available through three database vendors: Ovid, Dialog & DataStar <www.healthindex.com>* 2000

- *National Center for Chronic Disease Prevention & Health Promotion (NCCDPHP)* 1999

- *National Clearinghouse on Child Abuse & Neglect Information Documents Database* 1996

- *NIAAA Alcohol and Alcohol Problems Science Database (ETOH)* 1996

- *Psychological Abstracts (PsycINFO)* 1998

- *Referativnyi Zhurnal (Abstracts Journal of the All-Russian Institute of Scientific and Technical Information-in Russian)* 1996

- *Social Services Abstracts <www.csa.com>* 1996

- *Social Work Abstracts* 1996

- *Sociological Abstracts (SA)* 1996

- *SOMED (social medicine) Database* 1996

- *Violence and Abuse Abstracts: A Review of Current Literature on Interpersonal Violence (VAA)* 1996

(continued)

Special Bibliographic Notes related to special journal issues (separates) and indexing/abstracting:

- indexing/abstracting services in this list will also cover material in any "separate" that is co-published simultaneously with Haworth's special thematic journal issue or DocuSerial. Indexing/abstracting usually covers material at the article/chapter level.
- monographic co-editions are intended for either non-subscribers or libraries which intend to purchase a second copy for their circulating collections.
- monographic co-editions are reported to all jobbers/wholesalers/approval plans. The source journal is listed as the "series" to assist the prevention of duplicate purchasing in the same manner utilized for books-in-series.
- to facilitate user/access services all indexing/abstracting services are encouraged to utilize the co-indexing entry note indicated at the bottom of the first page of each article/chapter/contribution.
- this is intended to assist a library user of any reference tool (whether print, electronic, online, or CD-ROM) to locate the monographic version if the library has purchased this version but not a subscription to the source journal.
- individual articles/chapters in any Haworth publication are also available through the Haworth Document Delivery Service (HDDS).

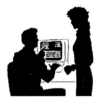

ABOUT THE EDITORS

Christopher B. Keys, PhD, is Professor of Psychology and Disability and Human Development and Chair of the Department of Psychology at the University of Illinois at Chicago. Dr. Keys is a past president of the Society for Community Research and Action and past Chair of the Council for Program Directors in Community Research and Action. The author of more than 100 publications and reports and over 250 presentations, Dr. Keys has been invited to lecture on his research in China, Australia, Europe and Latin America. Dr. Keys is interested in organizational and community processes that promote the empowerment of people with disabilities and their families. He and his colleagues have developed, implemented and evaluated interventions for developing disability advocates, establishing advocacy organizations, and building community coalitions on disability issues.

Peter W. Dowrick, PhD, is Affiliate Graduate Faculty member in Psychology, Professor of Disability Studies, and Graduate Studies in Psychology and has research interests in community-based programs that build creative futures and literacy development, especially in under-resourced areas. He directs multi-site projects in urban and rural Hawaii, urban Philadelphia, and Alaska. He is an international authority on using video in social and health sciences, especially in self-modeling and related uses of the "positive self-image," and has over 100 publications, including books, articles, and films. In the last 12 years, he has been Principal Investigator (PI) or Co-PI on over 35 grant-funded projects, with support from federal agencies, local government, and private foundations. A Fellow of the Society for Community Research and Action, he is founding Co-Chair of its Interest Group on Disability.

People with Disabilities: Empowerment and Community Action

CONTENTS

Community Psychology and Disability Studies   1
  Peter W. Dowrick
  Christopher B. Keys

Consumers as Collaborators in Research and Action   15
  Glen W. White
  Dorothy E. Nary
  A. Katherine Froehlich

Collaborative Ecological Community Interventions for People
  with Chronic Fatigue Syndrome   35
  Leonard A. Jason
  Amy M. Kolak
  Tonya Purnell
  Dan Cantillon
  Jennifer M. Camacho
  Susan Klein
  Allison Lerman

Empowering Latinos with Disabilities to Address Issues
  of Independent Living and Disability Rights:
  A Capacity-Building Approach   53
  Fabricio E. Balcazar
  Christopher B. Keys
  Yolanda Suarez-Balcazar

Community Responsiveness: Examples from Under-Resourced
  Urban Schools   71
  Peter W. Dowrick
  Thomas J. Power
  Patricia H. Manz
  Marika Ginsburg-Block
  Stephen S. Leff
  Soon Kim-Rupnow

Building Community Coalitions with People with Disabilities
    and Their Families: An Empowerment Approach   91
    Christopher B. Keys
    Alan R. Factor

Index   113

Community Psychology
and Disability Studies

Peter W. Dowrick

University of Hawaii at Manoa

Christopher B. Keys

University of Illinois at Chicago

SUMMARY. Both the field of community psychology and the disability rights movement, including the field of disability studies, have been growing over the last 30 years. While common values, principles, and strategies have emerged within these two fields, they have often emerged independently and in ignorance of each other. Recognition of the value of community psychology perspectives on disabilities and community action is the motivation both for this special volume and for the disability interest group of the Society for Community Research and Action. In this article, we examine the action steps different authors have identified as important in responding effectively to community needs. We identify a general model and three settings which require an adaptation of this general model. These settings differ in the extent to which the recipients (consumers, people with disabilities) are already established as a community, and the extent to which providers (agencies, government) have established relationships with that community. We offer concluding com-

---

Address correspondence to: Professor Peter W. Dowrick, Center on Disability Studies, 1776 University Avenue, UA4-6, or Professor Christopher B. Keys, Department of Psychology, MC 285, University of Illinois at Chicago, 1007 West Harrison Street, Chicago, IL 60607.

The editors appreciate the thoughtful, efficient assistance of Georgina Tegart in editing and organizing this special issue.

[Haworth co-indexing entry note]: "Community Psychology and Disability Studies." Dowrick, Peter W., and Christopher B. Keys. Co-published simultaneously in *Journal of Prevention & Intervention in the Community* (The Haworth Press, Inc.) Vol. 21, No. 2, 2001, pp. 1-14; and: *People with Disabilities: Empowerment and Community Action* (ed: Christopher B. Keys and Peter W. Dowrick) The Haworth Press, Inc., 2001, pp. 1-14. Single or multiple copies of this article are available for a fee from The Haworth Document Delivery Service [1-800-342-9678, 9:00 a.m. - 5:00 p.m. (EST). E-mail address: getinfo@haworthpressinc.com].

ments regarding collaboration and knowledge sharing between the field of disability studies and community psychology. *[Article copies available for a fee from The Haworth Document Delivery Service: 1-800-342-9678. E-mail address: <getinfo@haworthpressinc.com> Website: <http://www.HaworthPress.com> © 2001 by The Haworth Press, Inc. All rights reserved.]*

KEYWORDS. Disability studies, community psychology, disability rights movement, disability, community response models, action research

There are fifty-four million people in the U.S. who have been marginalized in society because of their disabilities (US Bureau of Census, 1999). Since the 1960s, with the advent of the disability rights movement and the emergence of the field of disability studies, there have been gradually increasing efforts to improve access and participation in the community for people with disabilities. In the same time span, the field of community psychology has emerged as the study of individuals and community systems, with increasing attention to the issue of the empowerment of members of marginalized groups. Surprisingly, these fields have evolved in parallel, with little interaction between the two.

A review of the current literature indicates that engagement between the two fields is lacking. Although scientist-activists who consider themselves community psychologists (including several authors in this issue) have published in disability journals (e.g., Balcazar, Keys & Garate-Serafini, 1995; Ward & Dowrick, 1997; White, Mathews & Fawcett, 1989), they have seldom showcased community psychology specifically. In addition, we find only twelve articles with disabilities as the primary content published in the last ten years in the four most commonly read US community psychology journals. The field of disability studies appears to have developed more from the impetus of education, health and applied behavior analysis than from community psychology, yet these two fields have developed common values, principles, and strategies independently of one another. This special volume highlights this underdeveloped opportunity for collaboration between disability studies and community psychology. Our primary focus here is first to provide a brief background on disability research and action and then to succinctly compare the approaches to community action with people with disabilities presented in this special collection.

DISABILITY RESEARCH AND ACTION

A consideration of the field of disability studies necessitates a consideration of the disability rights movement. The field of disability studies has both emerged from, and embodies the spirit of, the disability rights movement (Linton, 1998). The disability rights movement has become increasingly concerned with civil rights rather than with the development of services for people with disabilities (Gill, 1998). Its members have rejected approaches that focus on individual deficits and impairments, and have instead called attention to the social, cultural and political barriers and the frequent lack of fit between individual abilities and contextual demands faced by people with disabilities. A major outcome of the disability rights movement has been the (self) identification of people with disabilities as both a minority group and a marginalized group (Gill, 1998).

People with disabilities have historically been marginalized in education, employment, and community living. Most children with serious disabilities are given segregated education (US Department of Education, 1998). Only 26% of adults with severe disabilities (18-64 years of age) work full or part time (US Bureau of Census, 1997). Disproportionately few own their own homes (Prouty & Lakin, 1999; Braddock, Hemp & Parish, in press); disproportionately many are victims of abuse (Sobsey, 1994).

These conditions exist despite consistent progress in legislation and considerable improvements to services and life opportunities in the last 35 years. Far reaching statutes have been enacted in education, health, rehabilitation, research, advocacy, training, and community access. In 1963, a week before his death, President Kennedy signed into law an act (PL 88-164) that created a federally backed system to ensure service improvements, advocacy, and professional training related to "mental retardation," since re-authorized for "developmental disabilities" (Dowrick, 1998). In 1974, PL 94-142–sometimes known as the "Education of All Children Act"–prompted a new era in special education, with its underlying goal of inclusivity eventually giving rise to PL 105-17, the Individuals with Disabilities Education Act (IDEA) in 1997. The Rehabilitation Act of 1973 (PL 93-112 et seq.) was designed to improve employment and general living conditions for adults and children with disabilities. In 1990, the capstone to the disability civil rights movement, the Americans with Disabilities Act, mandated equal access to transportation, communication, shopping, entertainment, politics, adult education, . . . indeed to all opportunities of public life (PL 101-336 et seq.). The goal of these statutes and others (e.g., assistive technology legislation) is *independent living*, and is backed by advocacy groups including self-advocates, families, providers, and researchers.

Images of change are especially salient in the area of special education. Our terminology has moved from "mainstreaming" through "integration" to "full inclusion." And our images have moved from that of a rock with a stream swirling around it, through a cocoon of special instruction always in sight of potential peers, to a student genuinely sharing the trials and triumphs of curriculum in common with others with and without disabilities. The disabilities movement has promoted *people first* language on the basis of respect, not politics, and its members have sought the dignity of risk in ways that parallel the movements for equal opportunity across ethnicity and gender (Oliver, 1996).

The disability rights movement laid the groundwork for the development of the field of disability studies. Members of the disability movement and researchers realized both the necessity and value of the inclusion of the perspectives of people with disabilities in the research process. Current trends in disability studies research include: full engagement and involvement of research participants in the research process (Balcazar, Keys & Suarez-Balcazar, this volume), including involving people with disabilities as co-researchers (March, Steingold, Justice & Mitchell, 1997); the importance of choice-making and self-determination (Kearney & McKnight, 1997), and of self-advocacy and empowerment (Miller & Keys, 1996); the call for emancipatory research where researchers are made accountable to participants by opening their research up to scrutiny by participants (Stone & Priestly, 1996); and the need for continual methodological and conceptual innovations to face the challenge of doing research with a marginalized population (Raphael, Renwick & Brown, 1993). By definition, those who participate in disability studies research support the disability rights movement (Linton, 1993), and researchers therefore struggle with and seek to transcend the natural contentions between political and social action on the one hand, and scientific skepticism on the other.

The issues faced by people with disabilities and their allies are ones with which community psychologists and activists can resonate, because of their experiences with other marginalized groups. Community psychologists have long been concerned with "people in trouble" and with issues of empowerment. Rappaport (1981) characterized the changing views of "people in trouble" by community psychology as a movement away from an emphasis on deficits, to an emphasis on rights (concerned with access and barriers to access) and ultimately to an emphasis on empowerment (concerned with both needs and rights and with individuals' choice and control of their own lives). Community psychologists face issues similar to those faced by disability studies researchers regarding involvement by participants, the importance of context, the tension between scientific skepticism and social action, and the impact of the researcher on the research process.

The five articles in this volume are all concerned with community response to needs and focus on issues of empowerment, coalition building, and collaboration. They all highlight familiar community psychology principles and methods but also advocate unique approaches to research and action with members of a marginalized population. While the approaches, populations, and interventions are diverse, a general action model of community responsiveness can be extracted.

EMPOWERING COMMUNITY RESPONSE MODELS AND DISABILITY ISSUES

The overall pattern of impact of empowering community responses to disability issues, as modeled by all five articles in this volume, is as follows: *(1) people with disabilities having a voice; (2) people with expertise in generating resources assisting that voice; (1+2) creating action that makes an empowering difference in the lives of the original group of people.* The articles present effective action involving individuals of all ages (first grade students to senior citizens) and different ethnic groups (Latino, African-American, Caucasian, Vietnamese, Samoan, etc.), across a range of physical, cognitive, and health disabilities. The key elements of each approach are listed in Table 1. In three (Balcazar; Dowrick; Keys), the elements are explicit; in two (Jason; White) they are implied.

TABLE 1. Comparison of Major Steps in Community Action Indicated in Five Reports, Listed by First Author

General Model	Community Response Model (established communities of recipients and providers)	Coalition Building Model (communities of recipients and providers yet to be established)		Community Collaboration Model (communities of established recipients without relationships to providers)	
	Dowrick	Keys	Balcazar	White	Jason
Make entry connections	Community Expressed Needs	Leadership	Community Entry	Coalition	Team Development
Clarify roles and demonstrate commitment	Place established in Community System	Recruitment	Needs Identification	Questions Formed	Assessing Needs
Set goals and action plans	Working as a Resource	Collaborative Planning	Organizing in Community	Goal Setting	
Act collaboratively, get results	Building Community Capacity	Collaborative Action	Planning and Action	Determining Procedures/ Action	Collaboration
Monitor results, modify actions	Creating Positive Images		Monitoring Revisions	Examining Results	
Evaluate, disseminate, promote sustained activity	Participant Evaluations/ Data	Promotion, Sustenance of Activity	Sustenance	Validation and Dissemination	Evaluation and Sustenance

General Model

A general model of empowering community responsiveness can be distilled from these five approaches. This "bare bones," generalized model is made up of the following six steps:

1. Make entry connections.
2. Clarify roles and demonstrate commitment.
3. Set goals and action plans.
4. Act collaboratively, get results.
5. Monitor results, modify actions.
6. Evaluate, disseminate, promote sustained activity.

But such a "bare bones" model provides researchers with inadequate guidance for the successful empowerment of marginalized subcommunities. A workable model would require more strategies, from which a functional operation can be designed. Differences in the diversity of the participants do not contribute substantially to the differences of the five approaches. Rather, the underlying model must be individualized, in terms of operational details, to meet the differences in sub-communities, their pre-existing agendas and the relationships among their members. For example, the Dowrick et al. (this volume) model of *community responsiveness* differs from the Keys and Factor (this volume) model of *coalition building*, not because one is a school setting with children at risk for school failure and disability labels and the other concerns older adults with aging and disability issues. They differ on how established the community of interest is. The schools in which Dowrick and colleagues intervened are highly routinized social settings. The coalitions Keys and Factor build are being organized for the first time with no prior history as an intact social setting.

We have identified three kinds of settings that require special features to the model. These settings are differentiated by the extent to which the recipients (consumers, people with disabilities) are already established as a 'community,' and the extent to which the providers (agencies, government) have established relationships with that community. Thus we have delineated three adaptations of the generalized model:

a. A community response model, for established communities of recipients and providers.
b. A coalition building model, for communities of recipients and providers yet to be established.
c. A community collaboration model, for communities of established recipients without relationships to providers.

Community Response Model

The first adaptation, in a setting of established communities of recipients and providers, is exemplified in the description provided by Dowrick, Power, Manz, Ginsburg-Block, Leff, and Kim-Rupnow (this volume). In this approach, the community (school children) is in a well established relationship with the agency (the school, including the parents or other community members who come to work in the school setting). The essential and sometimes distinguishing strategies are noted to be:

- Only preliminary *'entry' connections* are required with established communities and agencies, although it is always by invitation. In common with other variations of the model, both needs and strengths are identified by the community. A Resource Team (community psychologists, etc.) assists the community with the design and implementation of the intervention. The needs and strengths assessment can usually be achieved earlier in this setting than in the other two.

- The job of *clarifying roles and demonstrating commitment* is separated into two phases. First, it is necessary to work out the Resource Team's place in the system relative to preexisting, usually well-established, roles. Second, commitment is demonstrated by making it very clear that the Resource Team is just that, a resource, and it is not present to manage, control, or otherwise disempower existing personnel. It is routinely difficult, but essential, for the Resource Team to hold back from doing what is easy, such as organizing an incentive system or a satisfaction survey, while building the self-sufficiency of communities or agencies. The resource function can also be demonstrated by providing extra help which is tangentially related to the project, such as recommending an expert specialist for a rare disorder.
- Working as a resource in this way, is also the most empowering opportunity to *set goals and action plans,* because it enables working within an established system without disrupting it.
- The next step is to *act collaboratively and get results.* The focus is on building capacity and responsibility within the community to achieve outcomes for which they can take ownership.
- Data are collected to *monitor results.* Staff and local community members are taught through capacity building to monitor themselves and each other, and to *modify their actions* and objectives where necessary.
- Finally, the Resource Team fosters the participatory ownership and publicizing of data-based outcomes, as part of the *evaluation and dissemination* step. That, combined with the identification of other resources, serves to *promote sustained activity* because of pride and investment in the achievements, and a potential willingness to see the value of reallocating internal resources.

A unique feature of the Dowrick model of community responsiveness is the emphasis on *positive visions,* a way of creating images of future success. This strategy may be just as valuable in other situations. It is increasingly emphasized throughout the last three steps identified in the general model.

Coalition Building Model

The second adaptation is necessary in a setting in which there are fewer pre-established relationships within the targeted community, and therefore insufficient community linkages with the agencies who might support its needs. There may also be multiple agencies and individuals that have few or tenuous relationships with each other. The adaptation is exemplified in the descriptions provided by Keys and Factor and by Balcazar, Keys, and Suarez-Balcazar (both in this volume) and concern the empowerment of adults with developmental disabilities and their families through coalition building and the empowerment of Latinos with disabilities using a capacity building approach.

The essential and distinguishing strategies are:

- In *making entry,* additional effort is needed to identify multiple leaders in sub-communities and different agencies. The identification of strengths and needs occurs later in the project, with additional time spent establishing relationships and communicating with key players.
- *Roles begin to be clarified* as partners are recruited at all levels in the system. An emphasis on empowering these partners to communicate effectively with each other and to make mutually important decisions is essential to *demonstrating the commitment* of both the research team and the other stakeholders.
- The *setting of goals and action plans* is achieved by spending the time to identify local needs, to lay out a long term agenda and to create a sense of organization within the community.
- To *act collaboratively and get results,* there is an emphasis in this model on the "chemistry of collaboration." That is, the basis for action requires fostering and teaching collaboration (both innovatively and by-the-book) where there are no established rules.
- The need *to monitor results and modify actions* is fulfilled in standard fashion, except as noted below with respect to 'empowerment.'
- A standard approach is sufficient *to evaluate and disseminate* the valued aspects of the project. Both articles describe an emphasis on efforts *to promote sustained activity* by creating a sense of ownership of relationships and outcomes (e.g., improved services, quality of life) that did not previously exist.

The special characteristic of these approaches in response to this second type of setting, is the emphasis on *empowerment* and what it means for marginalized people to take control of aspects of their lives and achieve valued outcomes. This strategy is important in addressing the challenges or barriers to achieving the steps identified in the general model.

Community Collaboration Model

The third adaptation occurs in a setting in which there is an identifiable, if loosely organized, community but a lack of identified, appropriate support by relevant agencies (cf. White, Nary and Froehlich, this volume; Jason et al., this volume). Their approaches concern people with physical disabilities and people with chronic fatigue syndrome.

The essential and sometimes distinguishing strategies are noted to be:

- Less effort is needed in *making entry* because of the existence of pre-established groups, although some care needs to be exercised in recognizing existing leadership and internal politics. The *identification of strengths and needs* can usually be achieved relatively quickly and early in the process, based partly on existing research.
- *Role clarification* is singularly important. Developing the collaborative team relationship between the community group and the resource team is one of the major tasks of this model. The resource team can *demonstrate commitment* in relatively simple ways, such as making the effort to meet the community group on its turf, or by providing new resources, such as the assistance of a student research assistant.
- The task of *setting goals and action plans* is driven by the recognition and refinement of existing goals. The resource team helps the community group determine effective procedures to meet these goals.
- To *act collaboratively and get results* is a natural extension of the above activities. Goals and procedures are determined collaboratively and the basis for action is not necessarily a separate step in this model.

- The need *to monitor results and modify actions* is fulfilled in standard fashion.
- A standard approach is sufficient *to evaluate and disseminate* the valued aspects of the project. Both the articles herein provide good examples of validating as well as *promoting sustained activity* by the participation in and ownership of the outcomes.

The special characteristic of these two approaches in response to this type of setting, is the emphasis on enabling the self-determination of consumers (in this case, people with disabilities) in the development of an action oriented coalition with a resource team (in this case, one which is university based).

CONCLUSIONS

A diverse range of projects, based on community psychology principles applied to disability issues, are presented in this special volume. It appears they have in common six major steps, but need further characterization to identify strategies of value. We have identified three settings that may account for essential differences in making specific applications effective. These settings differ with regard to the amount of prior organization and the existence of established relationships within the community of interest. We look forward to further analysis using a greater number of projects and perhaps identifying other sets of differentiating characteristics.

We believe the five articles presented here demonstrate the similarities between the field of disability studies and community psychology and are evidence of the great potential for collaboration between the two fields. All five articles fully embrace Kelly's notion of *constituent validity,* that "subjects" should become *participants,* and their perspectives should impact research from the initial planning stage through the evaluation stage (Keys and Frank, 1987). This notion, which developed as a guiding light in the field of disability studies (cf. Gill, 1998), is now considered vital to adventuresome community psychology research (e.g., Foster-Fishman & Keys, 1997). The research teams in this issue demonstrate not only a dedication and a commitment to overcoming the barriers to full involvement by research participants, they demonstrate the value and potential impact of such involvement. This involvement is considered critical to sustaining each of the interventions presented by the authors. Researchers in disability studies and community psychologists could enter a promising dialogue about overcoming obstacles to constituent validity in marginalized populations.

Like community psychologists, researchers in the field of disability studies struggle with the tension between academic and scientific skepticism, and the values of social action. The five articles presented here demonstrate diverse methodologies, both traditional (e.g., national surveys, experimental design) and adventuresome (e.g., participatory action research). In addition, many show a commitment to rigorous and consistent evaluation, both traditional (e.g., quantitative measures) and adventuresome (e.g., self-evaluation, consumer valued outcomes). These researchers also maintain a commitment to the principles of the disability rights movement and keep the perspective of people with disabilities central to their action research. We look forward to continual innovations as researchers in community psychology and disability studies grapple with the tensions between the need for rigorous methodology and the demands of social and political action.

In sum, these articles indicate that community action can be demystified and the road to improved quality of life for people with disabilities can be operationalized. Community psychologists are learning to adapt their approaches to work effectively with people with disabilities in different contexts, yet the same empowering goals and values are apparent across all these models. In the future, we hope that there will be more collaboration between the field of disability studies and community psychology. Such collaboration will expose disability studies scholars to valuable theory and research concerning community phenomena and give community psychologists a deeper understanding of the experience of disability.

REFERENCES

Balcazar, F.E., Keys, C.B., & Suarez-Balcazar, Y. (2001). Empowering Latinos with disabilities to address issues of independent living and disability rights: A capacity-building approach. *Journal of Prevention & Intervention in the Community, 21(2), 53-70.*

Braddock, D., Hemp, R., & Parish, S. (in press). *The state of the states in developmental disabilities: Final Report.* Chicago: Department of Disability and Human Development.

Dowrick, P.W. (1994). So what's a "University Affiliated Program" anyway? *Nursing Spectrum, 30(25), 12.*

Dowrick, P.W. (1998). A consideration of "Community Response Programmes" on disabilities or other issues of common concern. *New Zealand Journal of Psychology, 27*(2), 22- 27.

Dowrick, P.W., Power, T.J., Manz, P.H., Ginsburg-Block, M., Leff, S.S., & Kim-Rupnow, S. (2001). Community responsiveness: Examples from under-resourced urban schools. *Journal of Prevention & Intervention in the Community, 21(2), 71-90.*

Gill, C. (1998, Spring) Disability Studies: Looking at the FAQs. *Alert: The Newsletter of the Institute of Disability and Human Development, 9*(3).

Jason, L.A., Kolak, A.M., Purnell, T., Cantillon, D., Camacho, J.M., Klein, S., & Lerman, A. (2001) Collaborative ecological community interventions for people with Chronic Fatigue Syndrome. *Journal of Prevention & Intervention in the Community, 21(2), 35-51.*

Keys, C., & Factor, A. R. (2001). Building community coalitions with people with disabilities and their families: An empowerment approach. *Journal of Prevention & Intervention in the Community, 21(2), 91-112.*

Keys, C., & Frank, A. R. (1987). Community psychology and the study of organizations. A reciprocal relationship. *American Journal of Community Psychology, 15,* 239- 251.

Linton, S. (1998). *Claiming disability: Knowledge and identity.* New York: New York University Press.

National Association on Disabilities. (1998). *1998 N.O.D./Harris survey of Americans with disabilities.* Washington, DC: Louis Harris.

Oliver, M. (1996). *Understanding disability: From theory to practice.* New York: St Martin's Press, Inc.

Prouty, R., & Lakin, K. C. Eds. (1999) *Residential services for persons with developmental disabilities: Status and trends through 1998.* Minneapolis: University of Minnesota, Research and Training Center on Community Living, Institute on Community Integration.

Public Law 88-164. (1963). *Construction of university affiliated facilities for the mentally retarded.* Washington, DC: US Congress.

Public Law 93-112 (1973). *Rehabilitation Act.* Washington, DC: US Congress.

Public Law 94-142 (1974). *Education for All Handicapped Children Act.* Washington, DC: US Congress.

Public Law 101-336. (1990). *Americans with Disabilities Act.* Washington DC: US Congress.

Public Law 105-17. (1997) *Individuals with Disabilities Education Act.* Washington DC: US Congress.

Sobsey, R. (1994). *Violence and abuse in the lives of people with disabilities: The end of silent acceptance?* Baltimore, MD: Paul H. Brookes Publishing Co.

U.S. Bureau of the Census. (1999). *Americans with Disabilities: Statistical Brief.* Washington DC: US Department of Commerce.

US Bureau of Census. (1995) *Survey of Income and Survey Participation.* Washington, DC: US Department of Commerce.

U.S. Department of Education. (1998) *Annual Report to Congress on the Imple-mentation of The Individuals with Disabilities Education Act.* Washington DC: Department of Education.

White, G.W., Nary, D.E, & Froelich, A.K. (2001). Consumers as collaborators in research and action. *Journal of Prevention & Intervention in the Community, 121 (2), 15-34.*

Consumers as Collaborators in Research and Action

Glen W. White
Dorothy E. Nary
A. Katherine Froehlich

University of Kansas

SUMMARY. This paper discusses the role of consumers as collaborators in disability research conducted in the community. A comprehensive model of participatory action research is described and illustrated with research and training projects conducted in a collaborative arrangement between researchers and a Consumer Empowered Team. The paper describes how adherence to the model could be conducted in actual research and training settings and produce outcomes valued by the consumers at whom the interventions were targeted. The advantages and caveats to using the consumer as collaborator approach are discussed. *[Article copies available for a fee from The Haworth Document Delivery Service: 1-800-342-9678. E-mail address: <getinfo@haworthpressinc.com> Website: <http://www.HaworthPress.com> © 2001 by The Haworth Press, Inc. All rights reserved.]*

Address correspondence to: Glen W. White, PhD, Department of Human Development and Family Life, University of Kansas, 4001 Dole Human Development Center, Lawrence, KS 66045 (E-mail: Glen@ukans.edu).

The research in these case examples was supported by the National Institute on Disability and Rehabilitation Research (Grant H133B30012-96) and the Paralyzed Veterans of America, Education and Training Foundation (ETF 274-95).

The authors thank all the consumers with disabilities who have helped to shape our research to allow the resulting outcomes to be more relevant to their lives. They also thank Richard Gutierrez for his assistance with this manuscript.

[Haworth co-indexing entry note]: "Consumers as Collaborators in Research and Action." White, Glen W., Dorothy E. Nary, and A. Katherine Froehlich. Co-published simultaneously in *Journal of Prevention & Intervention in the Community* (The Haworth Press, Inc.) Vol. 21, No. 2, 2001, pp. 15-34; and: *People with Disabilities: Empowerment and Community Action* (ed: Christopher B. Keys, and Peter W. Dowrick) The Haworth Press, Inc., 2001, pp. 15-34. Single or multiple copies of this article are available for a fee from The Haworth Document Delivery Service [1-800-342-9678, 9:00 a.m. - 5:00 p.m. (EST). E-mail address: getinfo@haworthpressinc.com].

KEYWORDS. Participatory action research, collaboration, physical disabilities, focus groups, consumer-valued outcomes

CONSUMERS AS COLLABORATORS IN RESEARCH AND ACTION

Great discoveries and improvements invariably involve the cooperation of many minds. I may be given credit for having blazed the trail but when I look at the subsequent developments I feel the credit is due to others rather than to myself.

–Alexander Graham Bell

Participatory Action Research (PAR), what is it? Whyte (1991) states that "Participatory Action Research is *applied* research," but unlike traditional applied research, PAR encourages people in the organization or community under study to actively participate with the research scientist throughout the entire research process–from beginning to end (p. 20). One of the identifying features of PAR is that it empowers participants who are likely to be the targets of the research to have a partnership in shaping the research process (Yeich & Levine, 1992). Santelli, Singer, DiVenere, Ginsberg, and Powers (1998) posit that the action research approach elevates participants to a co-researcher role based on their insider status and local knowledge. This role suggests that participants, whether workers in a factory or people with disabilities in the community, are valued as experts based on their past history and experiences with the research issue or problem that is being addressed.

Thus, the researcher takes the role of learner to better understand participants' experiences. Some researchers view such collaboration as inefficient and costly, while others invite and use PAR to develop more relevant and rigorous research outcomes. These researchers support the assertion that PAR enhances the quality of the research process, including problem and hypothesis formulation (Greenwood, Whyte, & Harkavy, 1993), assistance with participant recruitment, and direction for data analyses on identified factors (Santelli et al., 1998).

PAR has been used by researchers in numerous areas including cooperative living (Whyte, Greenwood, & Lazes, 1989), community health initiatives (Fawcett et al., 1996; Schwab, 1997), cultural research (Chataway, 1997; Lykes, 1997), and self-help groups (Chesler,

1991). In addition, PAR has been used to better understand various disability populations such as persons with psychiatric disabilities (Rogers & Palmer-Erbs, 1994), families with children with disabilities (Santelli et al., 1998), persons with developmental disabilities (Gilner & Sample, 1993), and adults with physical disabilities (White, Nary, & Gutierrez, 1997). There is a growing literature on PAR (Bartunek, 1993; Heller, 1993), its basic principles (Fawcett, 1991; McTaggart, 1991), and how it can be implemented (Balcazar, Keys, Kaplan, & Suarez-Balcazar, 1998).

This paper presents and discusses a model for participatory action research, and it examines two case illustrations in which participants with various disabling conditions were invited to be involved in research studies at our Research and Training Center on Independent Living (RTC/IL). The benefits of the model for people with disabilities can be generalized to other community groups.

A MODEL FOR PARTICIPATORY ACTION RESEARCH

Figure 1 illustrates a model, which identifies the pervasiveness of PAR throughout the research process. The research process is influenced by both external and internal consumer involvement. Specifically, this PAR model is composed of four main components: (a) external consumer influences, (b) internal consumer influences through the Consumer Empowered Team, (c) the research process, and (d) consumer-valued outcomes. Each of these components is presented in more detail below.

External Consumer Influence

The influence of consumers' needs is often substantial even before a related research project is begun. There has been a trend among policy makers and research funders, such as the National Institute on Disability and Rehabilitation Research (NIDRR), to develop PAR priorities.

Policy makers. Policy makers are often petitioned by special interest groups and individuals regarding hundreds of issues. The issues often represent ideas that may not even be on the policy maker's "radar screen." One consumer activist group, ADAPT (American Disabled for Attendant Programs Today) has used tactics to make their

FIGURE 1. An illustrative model of the Participatory Action Research process

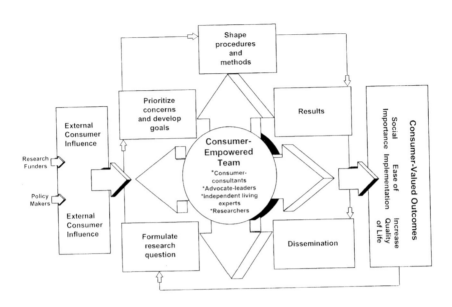

calls for change in policy widely publicized. ADAPT's campaign for accessible public transit began in Denver in 1983 and spawned 7 years of demonstrations in cities across the US. At those demonstrations wheelchair users blocked buses by chaining their wheelchairs to them. As a result, ADAPT was in a position to influence stringent requirements regarding public transit in the legislation of the *Americans with Disabilities Act 1990.*

Research funders. Funding agencies often solicit input when establishing research initiatives. Frequently the input is generated by professionals who wish to conduct research in the area. NIDRR is one such funding agency, which has initiated a system for assuring that this input comes not only from professionals, but also from consumers. Their consumer involvement approach has three components. First, they invite knowledgeable consumers, advocates, and family members of persons with disabilities to help identify real-world problems that need to be addressed through research. Second, in *The Federal Register,* they release "calls for public comment" on research priorities that they will incorporate in future grant competitions. Additional comments are directly solicited from disability advocates, families of children with disabilities, service providers, and researchers in the field. Third, NIDRR involves people with disabilities and those from minority cultures on its peer review panels for various grant competitions. While this process has some critics, it allows consumers to review the specified goals, procedures, and anticipated outcomes of proposed research projects. Consumers' comments provide a reality-check for the relevance of the proposed research, while the scientists on the panels provide input on the rigor of the proposed research.

Consumer Empowered Team

The Consumer Empowered Team (White, 1995), hereafter referred to as "the team," consists of consumer-consultants, advocate leaders, project independent living experts and researchers. The composition and design of the team is intended to produce project outcomes that are synergistic and mutually beneficial for participants and researchers. The team is much closer to research activities than the usual consumer advisory board. Its purpose is to solicit consumer input throughout the research process. Team composition varies depending on each project's goals. Team members may be recruited locally, regionally, or nationally. Consultations may range from interviewing key informants regarding policy issues, to developing contracts with subject matter experts to assist in producing specific research or training materials. The team is not a "one size fits all" approach, rather, each project assembles its own team based on the particular project needs, goals, and intended outcomes. The RTC/IL reimburses team members for their time and expenses, as would be done with any other group of experts.

Team members' perspectives help identify critical considerations of the proposed research. For example, team members frame the research issue from a consumer viewpoint, identify possible root causes of why the problem occurs, under what conditions, and with what consequences. Fawcett (1991) suggests this PAR process enhances the quality of the research process by assessing the social significance of the research *goals*; the appropriateness of the research *procedures*; and the social importance of the *effects* of the intervention.

The Research Process

The process starts with formulating the research question (Figure 1). To answer this question, the research goals, procedures and methods are developed. The generated data are then analyzed to identify the results and the results and intervention package, as applicable, are disseminated to targeted audiences. Each of these research elements and how they are influenced through this iterative participatory research process are discussed in more detail below.

Formulate research question. The team reviews and helps shape the research question within the priorities identified by the funding agency. This participation helps ensure that the research will be relevant to its intended targets. The iterative nature of the process naturally generates new research questions from the original question.

Prioritize concerns and develop goals. Within the direction of the research, the consumers' disability concerns are prioritized and goals developed to address those concerns. The team shapes the relevance of the concerns and goals based on their personal experience, by framing the particular problem being addressed in the research question. To provide general direction for our research issues and goals, the RTC/IL developed a Consumer Concerns Report Method (Schriner & Fawcett, 1988), which has been used to gather specific information on disability concerns from people with physical disabilities (Suarez de Balcazar, Bradford, & Fawcett, 1988).

Shape procedures and methods. Researchers adopt specific approaches to address research questions or problems. While the procedures used may embody rigorous methodology, sometimes they are contrived and unlikely to maintain the desired behavior or outcomes once the research is completed. As researchers, we desire to develop research interventions and outcomes which can survive in the natural community setting over time. The team teaches us valuable lessons about the delicate balance between research rigor and relevance. Rigorous research may be helpful in building science, but if it is not relevant to those to whom it is directed, it is unlikely to be adopted (Rogers & Palmer-Erbs, 1994).

Results. Traditional research results describe the effects of independent variables on targeted dependent variables and how this evidence contributes to existing knowledge. The main emphasis is whether the results have statistical significance or demonstrate a functional relationship between the independent and dependent variables. In a PAR approach, the team can augment the scientific interpretation of the results by challenging researchers to examine the practical meaning and impact the results can have for the targeted population. Consumer-collaborators will have little enthusiasm for research results that produce significant statistical effects, but have virtually no real-life application. Greenwood et al. (1993) state that this involvement in the research process is "capable of producing both scientifically and socially meaningful research results" (p. 180).

Dissemination. Consumer collaboration in the dissemination process can shape the products that flow from the research as well as the best formats (e.g., audiotape, Braille, large print, www, etc.) to promote maximum use by intended users. Consumer-collaborators who are partners in the research process can be valuable champions in approaching new target audiences for the particular intervention or resulting research products.

Consumer-Valued Outcomes

Consumers can also provide realistic input regarding research products through their perspective of the social importance of the outcomes, the ease of implementation, and whether outcomes improve some aspect of the consumers' quality of life. Each of these values is briefly discussed.

Social importance. Wolf (1978) and Fawcett (1991) have described the importance of consumer validation or social validation of research goals and procedures. These authors further suggest that consumer input is also relevant in determining the social importance of the effects of the research intervention and how relevant it is to their lives.

Ease of implementation. Consumers can provide a perspective that researchers, who are "on the outside," do not have about developing interventions that can be easily implemented by consumers. After the research phase has been conducted, emphasis should be placed on technology transfer from the researcher to the consumer, as recommended in the Institute on Medicine Report, *Enabling America* (Brandt & Pope, 1997).

Quality of life. Quality of life is an important issue to consumers when evaluating research interventions and proposed products. The following example highlights the significance of this issue. A rehabilitation researcher could develop a device to help a person with quadriplegia dress independently; however, the energy and time expended to dress may leave the person physically exhausted for the rest of the day. While the device is effective in assisting the person with quadriplegia get dressed, the energy exerted outweighs the benefits of dressing independently. Consumers' input is needed throughout the research process to increase the likelihood that research outcomes enhance consumers' quality of life.

Note that the Consumer-Valued Outcomes box in Figure 1 has an arrow that returns back to the formulation of new research questions. Ideally, the feedback from Consumer-Valued Outcomes could inform almost any level of the research cycle, thus creating an iterative process and program of research.

The next section describes two case illustrations in which participants with various disabling conditions were invited to be involved with projects conducted at the RTC/IL. To demonstrate the flexibility of the PAR process, we describe both a research study and a training package, developed in collaboration with consumers. The first illustration is on the development and empirical testing of an advocacy letter-writing package, *The Action Letter Portfolio* (White, Thomson, & Nary, 1999). The second is the development of resource booklets for people with spinal cord injuries on how to prevent or reduce the incidence of specific secondary complications.

Action Letter Portfolio

During the last 30 years, the US Congress has passed many laws to establish and protect the rights of citizens with disabilities. The most far-reaching legislation is the landmark civil rights law, the Americans With Disabilities Act of 1990 (ADA) (P.L. 101-336), which protects the rights of over 54 million citizens with disabilities (McNeil, 1997) in the areas of employment, public and private accommodations, and telecommunications. Despite passage of the ADA and other disability legislation, however, people with disabilities frequently struggle with discrimination and unfair treatment. One major reason is that fiscal and human resources for enforcing the regulations are limited. Therefore, it is important for citizens with disabilities to learn about the laws that protect them and to gain advocacy skills to promote compliance with these laws.

One social technology developed to meet this need is the Action Letter Portfolio, a self-administered training tool developed to help people with disabilities improve their advocacy letter writing skills. The Action Letter Portfolio outlines the components and methods of writing an action (or advocacy) letter, and provides examples and opportunities for manual users to practice these skills as they learn them. Users can also compare their letters with exemplars included in the manual. Both content (e.g., introduction to the problem, stating a rationale, providing evidence) and form (inside address, salutation, closing) are taught as essential elements of an effective advocacy letter. The manual provides information on targeting the letter to the proper recipient and on following up with recipients after letters are written. It also contains a section summarizing specific disability laws that can be cited in the letters as supporting information and evidence.

The development of this research project is described using the PAR model. The idea for the manual was conceived by a researcher with a disability as a result of personal frustration in trying to write a letter to an insurance company to advocate for a wheelchair more durable and lightweight than the guidelines allowed.

Team Composition

The team consisted of two nationally recognized disability advocates, one person with a severe physical disability, three researchers (two of whom had a disability), and a focus group of consumers who received the Action Letter materials as they were developed. Team members were chosen based on their ability and willingness to participate on this project.

Formulate the Research Question

The team conducted a literature search for exemplary materials. While training materials on letter writing to editors and public officials were found (Seekins, Fawcett & Mathews, 1987), these items were basic and lacked examples that addressed problems experienced by people with disabilities.

To learn more about what disability advocates and independent living experts were already doing in this area, the team sent a brief questionnaire to each center for independent living in the United States. Respondents were asked to identify the types of advocacy they presently used. Twenty-six percent of those independent living centers or programs responding to the questionnaire indicated that writing letters was their most frequent method used for advocacy.

Prioritize Concerns and Develop Goals

The survey also requested respondents to identify specific issue areas where advocacy training should be developed. Experts identified

14 different topics as critical for advocacy efforts. These topics included: (a) employment, (b) accessible parking, (c) disability policy, (d) public access, (e) transportation, (f) housing, (g) special services, (h) health care, (i) education, (j) insurance issues, (k) telecommunications, (l) media portrayal of people with disabilities, (m) vocational rehabilitation services, and (n) personal assistance services. These topics provided the team direction in obtaining specific US laws and regulations related to the selected areas (e.g., housing, and the Fair Housing Amendments Act of 1988). Summaries and key points of these laws were then included in the reference section of the Action Letter Portfolio materials.

Shape Procedures and Methods

The team met and discussed personal approaches to advocate for personal disability concerns they experienced, and to review the literature on different advocacy approaches. After much deliberation the team decided that teaching advocacy letter writing skills to consumers was the best course for this project. There were several reasons why this approach was taken. First, letter writing was already being used by centers for independent living. Second, the training could be self-administered; and third, letters provide a permanent product of the consumer's interaction with the intended target of the letter. After this decision was made, the team made a nationwide request to centers on independent living, independent living programs, and consumer-consultants with disabilities to submit exemplary advocacy letters they had previously written. These letters were assigned to one of the 14 identified topic areas based on their content. Team members reviewed them to determine if they had face validity and were likely to produce change.

Consumer focus groups confirmed that teaching people how to write effective advocacy letters was a good idea. Consumers recognized that the advocacy letters would leave a "paper trail" as evidence for later actions concerning trends towards non-compliance or continued discrimination. Based on the above information, team members wrote a five-chapter manual to serve as a reference guide for writing action letters.

A draft of the manual was sent out for review to independent living experts and IL advocacy staff members who were identified as representative of those most likely to use the materials. Following the manual revisions, a study was conducted with participants recruited from a rural independent living center to investigate whether the manual could be used in a self-administered manner to teach the letter writing skills (White, Thomson, & Nary, 1997). This phase incorporated consumer feedback by encouraging participants to record directly in their manuals any questions, ideas for improvement, or suggestions for the next revision of the manual.

Results

This multiple baseline across-participants study showed that ALP had modest effects with three of the four participants, indicating that individuals with no experience in writing advocacy letters can acquire these skills through use of a self-administered manual. While these participants increased the number of required elements in their letters, an error analysis indicated that participants frequently showed more improvement in the mechanical elements of the letters (e.g., date, opening salutation, and address) than in the content elements of the body of the letter (e.g., explanation of the personal disability concern, and rationale for the concern). These results taught the team that mastering the "content" sections of an advocacy letter may require more practice than the mechanical elements.

In a second study, three of the five participants showed moderate improvement in their advocacy letter-writing skills. While members of this group appeared to have difficulty generating personal disability concerns, once they did so, the letters based on these concerns scored higher than those based on hypothetical situations provided by researchers. This finding suggests that participants are likely to be better invested in writing an advocacy letter under more natural conditions.

Dissemination

Team members collaborated with other centers for independent living to do a national presentation of the Action Letter Portfolio as one tool that can be used as part of an overall advocacy strategy. The team discussed appropriate dissemination strategies in order to reach the largest number of consumers. The annual national independent living conference was suggested as an ideal mechanism to disseminate the ALP, since several hundred disability advocates usually attend. Information on the ALP has been disseminated in a product catalog and web page specifically targeted toward disability organizations.

There is strong evidence that there is interest in the ALP as a standing reference tool. Based on our original survey to centers for independent living that asked potential respondents, "Would your center purchase an advocacy letter training manual if one were available?" the great majority of responses (86%) indicated they would purchase an advocacy letter-writing manual.

Consumer-Valued Outcomes

In order to prompt consumer feedback about ALP's social importance, ease of implementation, and effect on the consumer's quality of life, each ALP manual includes an evaluation feedback form so that users can provide input regarding revisions for future editions. This information will also help shape new research questions in the area of enhancing consumer advocacy skills and approaches. Given the strong emphasis on advocacy in centers for independent living (Pope & Tarlov, 1991; White, Seekins & Gutierrez, 1996), we believe that this tool for social and community change will be well accepted by its intended users.

Social importance. Advocacy is one of the key components of consumer-run centers for independent living. Most centers have advocacy as one of their "core" services for consumers. Sixty-two percent of the centers responding to the survey reported having an advocacy group, however, they indicated that less than one-third of the consumers they work with have effective advocacy skills. This suggests that a training manual, such as ALP, might be of high importance for consumers to refer to and use when advocating for a personal disability concern.

Ease of implementation. This self-administered format allows centers for independent living staff the choice of conducting formal training or encouraging consumers to self-learn the materials. In addition, as designed, the ALP can serve as a reference manual that staff and consumers can use whenever they need to write advocacy letters.

Quality of life. Consumers have used the ALP to successfully advocate for change at the individual level and at the systems level. One notable example was a series of letters written to an international airport administration about the non-compliance of restroom facilities with current Americans With Disabilities Act Accessibility Guidelines. Following the instructions and examples outlined in the ALP, the consumer wrote advocacy letters that eventually convinced the airport administration to spend over $900,000 renovating each of its restrooms to exceed current federal accessibility requirements. Removing barriers to bathroom access is one important example of how using the ALP can increase consumers' overall quality of life.

To further illustrate the flexibility of the PAR process, we now turn to a training project designed to help people with disabilities to prevent or manage secondary health conditions.

Developing Resources for Preventing and Managing Secondary Conditions

People with disabilities are often at risk for other disabling problems. Pope and Tarlov (1991) call these problems secondary conditions, defined as health problems "causally related to a primary disabling condition" (p. 214). Health problems that can be secondary conditions include, but are not limited to: urinary tract infections, pressure sores, autonomic dysreflexia, spasticity, contractures, depression, chronic pain, upper-extremity problems, bowel problems, deconditioning and weight gain, syringomyelia, sleep disorders, heterotopic ossification, renal disease/failure, poor cardiorespiratory function, and orthostatic hypotension (Graitcer & Maynard, 1991).

External Consumer Influence

Paralyzed Veterans of America (PVA) provides roughly $500,000 per year for training grants submitted to its Spinal Cord Injury Education and Training Foundation. The priorities for training grants are usually developed by the board of directors, most of whom have a spinal cord injury or dysfunction. This board also responds to the PVA membership, all of whom have some type of spinal injury or dysfunction. Thus, there is a strong consumer influence on the training priorities before they are ever released for grant competitions. In fact the ETF grant submission guidelines require that proposals submitted must involve people with disabilities as part of the grant and project planning process.

Team Composition

The team consisted of nine topic experts in the area of secondary conditions. Six researchers (four of whom had a physical disability) and three consumers who either had, or were at risk of having, a secondary condition. Team members were chosen based on their ability and willingness to serve on this project.

Formulate the Research Question

For the purposes of this training, team members determined the specific training needs to help people with spinal cord injuries to prevent and manage secondary conditions. The team decided to develop resource materials–written in terminology consumers could understand–about preventing and managing specific secondary conditions.

Prioritize Concerns and Develop Goals

In 1992, the Research and Training Center on Independent Living received a grant from the Education and Training Foundation to develop and disseminate these materials. Development and prioritization of the materials was based on consultation with people at risk for secondary conditions to learn (a) which secondary conditions should be priorities, (b) what personal strategies consumers use to prevent or manage secondary conditions, and (c) which dissemination strategies should be used to target relevant audiences.

The first step was to convene a focus group of consumers who experienced a variety of motor-sensory disabilities and who were at risk for secondary conditions. The group focused on consumers' information concerning the frequency of secondary conditions and their costs, both in terms of medical treatment and time away from activities or isolation from society. This information helped the team shape a survey to gather data regarding the incidence and consequences of secondary conditions. The survey was randomly distributed nationally to over 400 consumers with physical disabilities. The survey results identified 12 secondary conditions of most concern to responders: (a) pressure sores, (b) urinary tract infections, (c) chronic pain, (d) chronic fatigue, (e) joint problems, (f) SCI and aging, (g) spasticity, (h) contractures, (i) deconditioning and (j) weight gain, (k) depression, (l) bowel dysfunction, and (m) sleep disturbance. Upon consultation with Hispanic PVA members, this last category was replaced with sexuality issues, due to the strong need for this information–and lack of it–in their culture.

Shape Procedures and Methods

The team then devised a system to incorporate consumer input into every step of the production of a booklet on each of these secondary condition topics. The process began with a literature search of over 100 articles from medical, health, and psychological databases for information on the specific topic. This information was synthesized, developed into an outline, and reviewed by the team for completeness and logic. From this outline, an editor wrote a 16-26 page resource booklet in consumer-friendly language for each of the twelve secondary topics.

A consumer focus group consisting of nine consumers with varying physical disabilities reviewed the draft manuscript and provided feedback on the accuracy, completeness, and readability of each booklet. Focus group members also contributed information from their personal experiences with secondary conditions, and management techniques they developed. For example, one member noted that there was an increased risk of pressure sores for pregnant women with spinal cord injuries who used wheelchairs because of the extra weight added to their body frame. This helpful tip prompted researchers to highlight the need for frequent pressure relief exercises for pregnant women who are wheelchair users.

Subject matter experts also reviewed the manuscripts. These individuals, many of whom were also people with disabilities, had national reputations for expertise in their disciplines. They provided an additional dimension of consumer input to the project.

Results

The results of this process were two-fold. First, a 2-page camera-ready newsletter insert with information about each specific secondary condition was produced. Many disability organizations communicate through newsletters, therefore an insert on each topic was provided to each organization to complement the more detailed resource booklets. The newsletter inserts encouraged readers to contact the disseminating organization for further information about secondary conditions and provided an additional opportunity for consumer input. Each insert solicited personal tips from consumer readers to assist others on how to prevent or manage secondary conditions. Submitters were paid $40 for each tip used in later newsletter inserts. The second product was a resource booklet on each of the identified secondary condition topics. These resource booklets were intended to be used in the organizations' libraries for direct consumer use in centers for independent living, Paralyzed Veterans of America chapters, and National Spinal Cord Injury Association chapters.

Dissemination

The team targeted the above organizations as dissemination points of the developed materials. Additionally, these products were promoted in the Research and Training Center's material catalogs and Internet home page, and PVA's national magazine *Paraplegia News.*

Through the multiplicative effects of newsletter distribution and distribution through other sources, the potential readership for these materials was estimated to be approximately 400,000 to 500,000 readers per secondary condition topic. Initially, all publications were written in English. However, after reviewing the incidence and prevalence of injury among Hispanic people, and consulting with Hispanic PVA members, the team approached PVA's Education and Training Foundation (ETF) to fund translation and publication of each of the secondary condition resource booklets in Spanish. After receiving ETF approval and funding, the booklets were written in Spanish by professional translators, and disseminated to Hispanic/Latino consumers with disabilities in Texas, Florida, California, New York, New Mexico, Mexico, Puerto Rico, and Peru.

Consumer-Valued Outcomes

Consumers have increasingly recognized that good health and prevention of secondary conditions is an important part of living independently (White et al., 1996). People with disabilities are more enthusiastic about taking personal control over their health than having medical professionals make decisions in "their best interest" (De-Jong, 1979).

Social importance. The incidence of secondary conditions for persons with disabilities is high. For the purposes of illustration we will use the secondary condition of pressure ulcers. Data show that over 60% of spinal injured patients in the Model SCI System Centers have had at least one pressure ulcer (Yarkony & Heinemann, 1995). The development of pressure ulcers may result in time away from work, extended periods of isolation (White, Mathews, & Fawcett, 1989), and loss of independence (White et al., 1996). Economically, the medical treatment for severe cases of pressure ulcers can cost as much as $90,000 per wound (Wharton, Milani, & Dean, 1987).

Ease of implementation. The materials were developed to be integrated with naturally occurring practices at targeted dissemination sites. The majority of the sites had a newsletter they regularly published. The camera-ready inserts called "Second Thoughts" were developed to fit in with most organizations' newsletters. The accompanying resource booklets were designed to be incorporated into each organization's library to be used as a reference tool by both staff and consumers.

Quality of life. As people with disabilities age, they are more vulnerable to the interactive effects of aging and onset of secondary conditions (Whiteneck et al., 1993). Consumers can incorporate the information and suggested behaviors contained in these materials to help postpone premature onset of secondary conditions which occur with the aging process. A decrease in frequency, severity, and duration of secondary conditions will promote a higher quality of life for consumers.

SUMMARY AND DISCUSSION

This paper illustrates the role of consumers as collaborators in community-based disability research and training. A comprehensive model of participatory action research was described with four primary components: external consumer influence, involvement of the Consumer Empowered Team, the research process, and consumer-valued outcomes. Illustrations of these components were provided by describing two research and training projects conducted by the Research and Training Center on Independent Living. These projects demonstrated how adherence to the model can be conducted in actual research and training settings. Additionally, these exemplars indicated how the team played a central role in shaping and amplifying the participatory action research process. The results from the identified research and training projects suggest that PAR helped produce outcomes that were valued by the consumers likely to benefit from the interventions.

Embracing the philosophy and practice of PAR is important for psychologists and others conducting research in the community. PAR enhances the trust relationship between the researchers and those being studied. Additionally, PAR allows consumer-collaborators a voice in the priorities of the research; in the goals, procedures, and outcomes of the research; and in how the results are disseminated. As professionals collaborate with consumers on research issues they gain real-life insights on the person-context factors that contribute to problems affecting people with disabilities.

While the PAR approach is increasingly discussed and used by researchers (Balcazar et al., 1998; Boyce, 1998; Krogh, 1998), it is not without concerns. For example, time needed to conduct research is increased as consumer-collaborators become involved. Collaboration also encourages researchers to develop research that is both rigorous and relevant. Sometimes that means justifying a specific research design or procedure to the team. Although the PAR approach may be more costly in terms of the increased numbers of individuals associated with a project, the argument can be made that PAR is cost effective because it shapes research interventions that are then actually used by their intended targets rather than simply appearing as publications in professional journals.

The great English philosopher and logician Bertrand Russell said, "Although this may seem a paradox, all exact science is dominated by the idea of approximation." Perhaps if we, as community psychologists, make enough successive approximations of what PAR should be, it will contribute to a more robust science, a more relevant science, and certainly a more friendly and empowering science.

REFERENCES

Americans with Disabilities Act of 1990. P. L. 101-336.

Balcazar, F. E., Keys, C. B., Kaplan, D. L., & Suarez-Balcazar, Y. (1998). Participatory action research and people with disabilities. *Canadian Journal of Rehabilitation, 12*(2), 105-112.

Bartunek, J. M. (1993). Scholarly dialogues and participatory action research. *Human Relations, 46*(10), 1221-1233.

Boyce, W. (1998). Participation of disability advocates in research partnerships with health professionals. *Canadian Journal of Rehabilitation, 12*(2), 85-93.

Brandt, E. & Pope, A. (Eds.) (1997). *Enabling America: Assessing Rehabilitation Science and Engineering.* Washington, DC: Institute of Medicine, National Academy of Sciences.

Chataway, C. J. (1997). An examination of the constraints on mutual inquiry in a Participatory Action Research project. *Journal of Social Issues, 53*(4), 747-765.

Chesler, M. A. (1991). Participatory Action Research with self-help groups: An alternative paradigm for inquiry and action. *American Journal of Community Psychology, 19*(5), 757-768.

DeJong, G. (1979). Independent Living: From social movement to analytic paradigm. *Archives of Physical Medicine and Rehabilitation, 60,* 435-466.

Fawcett, S. B. (1991). Social validity: A note on methodology. *Journal of Applied Behavioral Analysis, 24*(2), 235-239.

Fawcett, S. B., Paine-Andrews, A., Francisco, V., Schultz, J., Richter, K., Lewis, R., Harris, K., Williams, E., Berkeley, J. Y., Lopez, C. M., Fisher, J. L. (1996). Empowering community health initiatives through evaluation. In D. Fetterman, S. J. Kaftanian, & A. Wandersman (Eds.), *Empowerment evaluation: Knowledge and tools for self-assessment and accountability* (pp. 161- 187). Thousand Oaks: Sage.

Gilner, J. A., & Sample, P. (1993). *Participatory action research: An approach to evaluate community integration for persons with developmental disabilities.* Paper presented at the Annual Meeting of the American Evaluation Association, Dallas, TX.

Graitcer, P. L., & Maynard, F. M. (Eds.). (1991). *First colloquium on preventing secondary disabilities among people with spinal cord injuries* (pp. 119-120). Atlanta, GA: U.S. Centers for Disease Control and Prevention.

Greenwood, D. J., Whyte, W. F., & Harkavy, I. (1993). Participatory Action Research as a process and as a goal. *Human Relations, 46*(2), 175-192).

Heller, F. (1993). Another look at action research. *Human Relations, 46*(10), 1235-1242.

Krogh, K. (1998). A conceptual framework of community partnerships: Perspectives of people with disabilities on power, beliefs, and values. *Canadian Journal of Rehabilitation, 12*(2), 123-134.

Lykes, M. B. (1997). Activist participatory research among the Maya of Guatemala: Constructing meanings from situated knowledge. *Journal of Social Issues, 53*(4), 725-746.

McTaggart, R. (1991). Principles for participatory action research. *Adult Education Quarterly, 41*(3), 168-187.

Pope, A. M., & Tarlov, A. R. (1991). *Disability in America: Toward a national agenda for prevention.* Washington, DC: National Academy Press, Institute on Medicine.

Rogers, E. S., & Palmer-Erbs, V. (1994). Participatory Action Research: Implications for research and evaluation in psychiatric rehabilitation. *Psychosocial Rehabilitation Journal, 18*(2), 3- 12.

Santelli, B., Singer, G. H. S., DiVenere, N., Ginsberg, C., & Powers, L. E. (1998). Participatory Action Research: Reflections on critical incidents in a PAR project. *JASH, 23*(3), 211-222.

Schriner, K. F., & Fawcett, S. B. (1988). Development and validation of a community concerns report method. *Journal of Community Psychology, 16*, 306-316.

Schwab, M. (1997). Sharing power: Participatory public health research with California teens. *Social Justice, 24*(3), 11-29.

Seekins, T., Fawcett, S.B., & Mathews, M. (1987). Effects of self-help guides on three consumer advocacy skills: Influencing public policy. *Rehabilitation Psychology, 32*, 29-38.

Suarez de-Balcazar, Y, Bradford, B., & Fawcett, S. B. (1988). Common concerns of disabled Americans: Issues and options. *Social Policy, 19*, 29-35.

Wharton, G. W., Milani, J. C., & Dean, L. S. (1987). Pressure sore profile. *Proceedings of the American Spinal Cord Injury Association*, 115-119.

White, G. W. (1995). *Consumer involvement in the research process: Balancing research relevance with research rigor.* Paper presented at the National Institute on Disability and Rehabilitation Research Project Director's Meeting, Washington, DC.

White, G. W., Mathews, R. M., & Fawcett, S. B. (1989). Reducing risk of pressure sores: Effects of watch prompts and alarm avoidance on wheelchair push-ups. *Journal of Applied Behavior Analysis, 22*(3), 287-295.

White, G. W., Nary, D. E., & Gutierrez, R. G. (1997). *Tools for empowerment for persons with disabilities using individual, group and community engagement.* Paper presented at the 6th Biennial Conference on Community Research and Action, Columbia, SC.

White, G. W., Seekins, T., & Gutierrez, R. (1996). Preventing and managing secondary conditions: A proposed role for independent living centers. *Journal of Rehabilitation, 62*(3), 14-21.

White, G. W., Thomson, R., & Nary, D. E. (1997). An empirical analysis of the effects of a self-administered advocacy letter training program. *Rehabilitation Counseling Bulletin, 41*(2), 74-87.

White, G. W., Thomson, R., & Nary, D. E. (1999). *The Action Letter Portfolio.* Lawrence, KS: The Research and Training Center on Independent Living at the University of Kansas.

Whiteneck, G. G., Charlifue, S. W., Gerhart, K. A., Lammertse, D. P., Manley, S., Menter, R. R., & Seedroff, K. R., (Eds.). (1993). *Aging with spinal cord injury.* New York: Demos.

Whyte, W. F. (Ed.) (1991). *Participatory Action Research.* Newbury Park, CA: Sage.

Whyte, W. F., Greenwood, D. J., & Lazes, P. (1989). Participatory action research: Through practice to science in social research. *American Behavioral Scientist, 32*(5), 513-551.

Wolf, M. M. (1978). Social validity: The case for subjective measurement *or* how applied behavior analysis is finding its heart. *Journal of Applied Behavior Analysis,11*(2), 203-214.

Yarkony, G. M., & Heinemann, A. W. (1995). Pressure ulcers. In S. L. Stover, J. A. DeLisa, & G. G. Whiteneck (Eds.), *Spinal Cord Injury: Clinical outcomes from the model systems* (pp. 100- 119). Gaithersburg, MD: Aspen.

Yeich, S., & Levine, R. (1992). Participatory research's contribution to a conceptualization of empowerment. *Journal of Applied Social Psychology, 22*(4), 1894-1908.

Collaborative Ecological Community Interventions for People with Chronic Fatigue Syndrome

Leonard A. Jason
Amy M. Kolak
Tonya Purnell
Dan Cantillon
Jennifer M. Camacho
Susan Klein
Allison Lerman

DePaul University

SUMMARY. A key value of community psychology research is the collaborative relationship between researchers and the actual groups under study. This article provides an example of a long term, multidimensional, collaborative, and ecologically-oriented research and action approach. This collaboration involved researchers and students at an urban university and a self-help organization of patients diagnosed with chronic fatigue syndrome. Epidemiological research and needs assessments laid the foundation for advocacy and program development efforts. These efforts in turn gave rise to further, more focused research and evaluation. The social construction of knowledge and the initiation of social change from an ecological perspective best involves interdisciplinary and community collaboration. *[Article copies available for a fee from The Haworth Document Delivery Service: 1-800-342-9678. E-mail address: <getinfo@haworthpressinc.com> Website: <http://www.HaworthPress.com> © 2001 by The Haworth Press, Inc. All rights reserved.]*

Address correspondence to: Leonard A. Jason, PhD, Department of Psychology, DePaul University, 2219 North Kenmore, Chicago, IL 60613.

[Haworth co-indexing entry note]: "Collaborative Ecological Community Interventions for People with Chronic Fatigue Syndrome." Jason et al. Co-published simultaneously in *Journal of Prevention & Intervention in the Community* (The Haworth Press, Inc.) Vol. 21, No. 2, 2001, pp. 35-51; and: *People with Disabilities: Empowerment and Community Action* (ed: Christopher B. Keys and Peter W. Dowrick) The Haworth Press, Inc., 2001, pp. 35-51. Single or multiple copies of this article are available for a fee from The Haworth Document Delivery Service [1-800-342-9678, 9:00 a.m. - 5:00 p.m. (EST). E-mail address: getinfo@haworthpressinc.com].

KEYWORDS. Chronic Fatigue Syndrome, ecological model, advocacy, collaboration, mentor program, self-help groups

Kingry-Westergaard and Kelly (1990) have suggested that a fundamental principle of an ecological approach involves using multiple methods to understand complex qualities of relationships and systems. One of these methods for helping to understand what we claim to know is the collaborative relationship between the researcher and the participants. This means that concepts and hypotheses are developed and tested by both the researcher and the participants. In a sense, the ecological endeavor is a discovery process where the different parties share the different constructions of their contexts, learn of those events and processes that help define their understanding of the contexts, and work together to define the research activity. This mutually empowering, egalitarian and respectful relationship is a key aspect of community interventions (Serrano-Garcia, 1990).

Kelly (1986) has posited that ecological principles should be used by professionals who join in long-term collaborative relationships with persons and settings. By involving participants actively in the planning of interventions, the recipients of the programs receive support, learn to identify resources, and become better problem-solvers who are more likely to manage future problems and issues. Interventions that have been generated from collaboratively defined, produced, and implemented change efforts are more apt to endure. By involving participants in the design of the research, investigators might gain a greater appreciation of the culture and unique needs of the community, and heighten the possibilities of the research findings being used to benefit the community. An ecological approach would involve examining a community's basic values, and analyzing community traditions for responding to community problems. It also would include creating citizen advisory groups to gather community support and interpret the goals of an intervention, and assessing positive and negative second-order ripple effects of an intervention.

This paper uses this ecological model as a conceptual framework that orients a series of descriptive examples. We will target in this article those aspects of Kelly's ecological model that are most relevant to understanding the distinctive contributions of community psychology to a joint university-advocacy group effort and an interdisciplinary research collaboration. We will argue that the initiation of social change from an ecological perspective best involves interdisciplinary and community collaboration. Two questions addressed in this article are: (1) how can one initiate an ecologically-based response to deal with health problems caused by chronic fatigue syndrome (CFS) that severely interferes with individuals' quality of life, and (2) what are an ecological model's contributions to those interested in chronic fatigue syndrome (CFS).

Chronic fatigue syndrome (CFS) appears to be a heterogeneous disease syndrome that may be triggered by a variety of factors (Jason, Wagner et al., 1995). The most prominent symptom is persistent fatigue for at least 6 months. Other symptoms commonly reported include: mild fever or chills, sore throats, painful lymph nodes, unexplained generalized muscle weakness, muscle discomfort, prolonged generalized fatigue after levels of exercise, generalized headaches, joint swelling, neuropsychiatric complaints, and sleep disturbances. Relatively few patients recover, with most continuing to experience decreases in exercise tolerance and mild CFS-related symptoms which are exacerbated during periods of stress and minor illness (Wilson et al., 1994). While there are several theories of etiology of this syndrome, considerable controversy exists about the nature of the possible biological, psychological, constitutional and genetic contributory factors (Friedberg & Jason, 1997). This lack of agreed upon and established etiology presents researchers with a unique challenge: how to conduct research in a sensitive and comprehensive way, and not inadvertantly stigmatize those with this illness as having a "psychiatric illness."

When a new disease syndrome emerges, such as chronic fatigue syndrome, studies on etiology and prevalence can shape public policy. For example, the number of individuals identified with the syndrome may influence the federal and state resources allocated for research, prevention, and intervention (Friedberg & Jason, 1998). Community psychologists have key roles to play in epidemiologic research with new disease syndromes. The first generation of chronic fatigue syndrome epidemiologic studies were flawed because of their reliance upon physician referrals, resulting in findings that underestimated the prevalence of chronic fatigue syndrome and thus minimized the seriousness of this illness. In such a situation, community psychologists could participate in assembling multi-disciplinary teams to conduct more rigorously designed research that better estimates the prevalence of the syndrome. As a consequence, we could help set the agenda for how the epidemiologic research is conceptualized, which could influence the development of public policy.

DEVELOPING A RESEARCH TEAM

Beginning in 1991, Leonard Jason and Judy Richman began assembling a research team to work with individuals diagnosed with chronic fatigue syndrome. At the time, there were few services available for people with this illness, and many medical personnel were skeptical of its existence. Rather than attempting first to develop social or community interventions, we felt the most important objective was to conduct basic research into the prevalence of this syndrome. In the early 1990s, this disorder was considered a relatively rare condition, affecting less than 20,000 people in the US (Gunn, Connell, & Randall, 1993).

Our research team in Chicago included more than 15 professionals from diverse areas, including epidemiology, psychiatry, medicine, immunology, sociology, biostatistics, and community psychology. Members of the Chicago Chronic Fatigue Syndrome Association also actively participated in meetings where the methods of our studies were discussed. The group was united in gathering pilot chronic fatigue syndrome epidemiologic data from a random community sample, validating measurement approaches and instruments, and developing and securing a grant proposal to study the epidemiology of chronic fatigue syndrome in a large scale community sample (Jason, Wagner et al., 1995). Our initial findings indicated that over 400,000 people had current CFS in the US, a figure over 20 times higher than the official rates from the Centers for Disease Control (Jason, Taylor et al., 1995). This pilot work was used to secure a NIH grant involving a large community-based epidemiology study of CFS, which is currently ongoing. Our research with random community samples is now being used by other investigators, including those from the Centers for Disease Control. In an earlier project, we assessed the prevalence of CFS among nurses (Jason et al., 1993), and the data from this study encouraged a nurse with CFS to form the organization called Medical Professionals/Persons with CFS (Gail Dahlen, Personal Communication, March 31, 1998). Bringing together scientists from different disciplines is a critical step in seeking a better understanding and more thorough investigation of complex disease entities and conditions.

When community psychologists address population issues that are not easily explained, such as chronic fatigue syndrome, we can advocate for research that avoids stigmatization potentially caused by biases and unexamined assumptions. In the chronic fatigue syndrome arena, key decisions were made within a socio-political context in which chronic fatigue syndrome was assumed to be a psychologically-based problem (Friedberg & Jason, 1997). Many physicians continue to believe that most individuals with the syndrome have a psychiatric illness. Due to the controversy surrounding chronic fatigue syndrome diagnoses, people with the syndrome frequently face disbelieving attitudes from their doctors, family and/or friends, and many experience profound losses in their support systems. One major consequence is that many people with chronic fatigue syndrome feel dissatisfied with their medical care and have gone outside traditional medicine to be treated for their illness (Jason, Ferrari, Taylor, Slavich, & Stenzel, 1996).

Vercoulen et al. (1996) provided an 18-month follow-up of 246 patients with CFS, finding that only 3% reported complete recovery and 17% reported improvement. It is possible that these discouraging follow-up statistics are in part due to the lack of effective supports available in the community to help recover (Ware & Kleinman, 1992). The key question concerns the types of changes that might be most important. Below, we review several large-scale surveys that have assessed the patients' perspectives.

NEEDS ASSESSMENT

To more effectively assess the needs of people with CFS, Jason, Ferrari, Taylor, Slavich, and Stenzel (1997) analyzed a brief survey of open- and closed-ended items designed to assess the participants utilization of and preference for a variety of services. The questionnaire consisted of fourteen 5-point (1 = undesirable; 5 = extremely desirable) rating scales. These items were developed with consultation from members of the Chicago Chronic Fatigue Syndrome Association. Respondents with CFS (n = 984) were instructed to indicate their preference for each of the 14 hypothetical rehabilitation services that might assist their recovery. This was the first survey of its kind distributed to a national sample of people with chronic fatigue syndrome. Advocacy services were the highest-rated factor–not surprising, given the discrimination and negative attitudes that people with this disorder endure. Preferred advocacy efforts included a telephone hotline service providing immediate advice and assistance on recovery, an advocacy worker to secure financial resources and legitimize the service needs of individuals with CFS, and a volunteer caregiver system to provide assistance with daily chores and errands. Respondents with CFS also made a strong plea for needed education within the medical field, government, and general public. Educational efforts would aim to increase knowledge regarding the legitimacy and existence of CFS as a disease entity. In turn, increased knowledge would increase the quality of medical care, financial resources, and services offered for individuals with CFS. The second-highest-priority items were self-help groups providing emotional support and current treatment information. This result is consistent with other studies indicating that individuals with CFS need continued social and emotional support to cope effectively with their illness.

These data helped set priorities for the subsequent development of service programs, as there were areas identified as having significant need (e.g., housing, jobs, volunteer buddies, etc.), but no services or programs were currently available to meet these needs. We did not need to create self-help groups or telephone hotlines, as these were already established within the Chicago metropolitan area.

A COLLABORATIVE RELATIONSHIP

In addition to learning about the needs from people with chronic fatigue syndrome nationally, our research team began building a collaboration with the local Chicago Chronic Fatigue Syndrome Association. We followed an ecological model in developing this relationship. Thus, the university personnel and self-help group members were equal parties in both the design and implementation of the interventions. Below, we report on a series of intervention pilot programs that address issues such as employment, housing, and daily assistance.

EMPLOYMENT

For many people with CFS, fatigue seriously interferes with work (Friedberg & Jason, 1998). Loss of work can be a devastating and demoralizing experience. Many people with CFS believe there is little hope of finding employment, particularly employment that has a flexible schedule. People with CFS may have more energy on some days than on others and no way of predicting his or her energy level. Flexibility at the work site is a key need for people with chronic fatigue syndrome in search of part-time employment (LeRoy, Davis, & Jason, 1996).

Most agencies still are not sure how to develop supportive programs for people with severe energy deficits. Because people with this syndrome often appear healthy when they come into service agencies seeking job counseling or other services, the service providers often do not understand that these individuals might only have a few hours each week to give to an employer. Full-time employment is not possible for most people with this syndrome. What is needed is job assessment, part-time job opportunities, support and encouragement, followed by a gradual increase in the number of hours devoted to work each day.

To deal with these employment issues more effectively, a member of the DePaul University research team and a group of people with chronic fatigue syndrome formed a part-time job committee to develop a job bank. This committee was a collaborative DePaul University-Chicago Chronic Fatigue Syndrome Association effort. This group was different from more traditional self-help groups, as the primary focus was on helping members discover job opportunities. The participants of the part-time job committee also attended the monthly self-help support meetings sponsored by the Chicago Chronic Fatigue Syndrome Association.

A well-known disability lawyer was invited to attend one of the meetings and share his knowledge in this area. He discussed eligibility requirements for obtaining social security benefits, and ways to transition into part-time job opportunities without losing medical and financial benefits of the social security disability program. The committee decided to create a job bank that would provide listings of part-time jobs that might be appropriate for people with chronic fatigue syndrome. Some home-based employment opportunities, such as multilevel marketing, proofreading, and home office computing, might allow people with chronic fatigue syndrome to set their own work schedules. The researcher and six people with chronic fatigue syndrome met on a monthly basis to locate and review part-time jobs and place them in the job bank.

The job committee gave members a chance to gain emotional support and encouragement while thinking about ways of rejoining the workforce on a part-time basis. The support group allowed participants to reduce their sense of isolation, to develop confidence, and to have a forum to discuss common problems (Maton, 1989). Several people were able to begin part-time house sitting, pet sitting, and telemarketing jobs. The job directory continues to be updated and is available to all the members of the Chicago Chronic Fatigue Syndrome Association. A key feature of this program is that it was developed with input and structure from both a member of the research team and members of the self-help group, and this collaborative relationship helped each party stay committed to the project.

We experienced many advantages in employing this type of ecological approach. By working cooperatively with members of the self-help community in planning the functions and activities of the job committee, our research team gained a better appreciation of the needs and talents of those in the self-help group, and the students appreciated the fact that our work was valued by the community members. In addition, these collaborative experiences helped the leadership of the CFS organization to develop high levels of trust with the DePaul University investigators, as they came to see them as allies who were interested in working cooperatively with them on the planning of new services. As one indication of this positive regard, the members of the Chicago Chronic Fatigue Syndrome Association nominated the first author to receive an award from the national CFS organization for outstanding support for people with CFS, and this award was presented to him in 1997.

HOUSING

Because people with chronic fatigue syndrome are often unable to work, many find themselves in danger of losing their housing (Davis, Jason, & Banghart, 1998). When people become very sick with chronic fatigue syndrome, many could profit from a setting or community to protect them so that their health can improve. At present, these types of treatment settings are not available for people with chronic fatigue syndrome.

We first sought input on housing initiatives through a survey distributed by a national newsletter for people with chronic fatigue syndrome (based on the survey described earlier, Jason et al., 1996). We collaborated with members of the Chicago Chronic Fatigue Syndrome Association in developing the items for this survey. Respondents indicated housing services were a moderately desirable need among people with chronic fatigue syndrome. Using 5-point (1 = undesirable; 3 = moderately desirable; 5 = extremely desirable) rating scales, our respondents gave average ratings of 3.5 to the statement: "Allowing a carefully-screened person to live in a person with chronic fatigue syndrome's home; the healthy person would help with errands, chores and provide support, and in return would have a place to live and a small stipend," and a rating of 3.4 to the item: "A referral service where people with chronic fatigue syndrome can find roommates to share housing," and a rating of 3.3 to the item: "An integrated home with people with chronic fatigue syndrome living on the bottom floor, college students on the second floor and a couple or family as the house managers; the student helpers would be assigned to help the people with chronic fatigue syndrome with errands, chores, and cooking, etc."

A shared housing program has the potential of providing an inexpensive place to live without dependence upon outside agencies or governmental programs. A shared housing program might involve others sharing their homes with people with chronic fatigue syndrome. During this time of state and federal funding cutbacks, developing programs that are financially independent and self-supporting is a high-priority goal. In addition, there is the obvious benefit of shared monthly expenditures for rent, utilities, and food. Also, people with chronic fatigue syndrome might save energy by sharing some household duties like cleaning and shopping, activities that can be overwhelming for people with chronic fatigue syndrome who live alone. In addition, emotional well-being can be increased by living with a sympathetic housemate who understands the illness and can provide support.

We have contacted various organizations and agencies that successfully implemented shared housing programs for elderly populations. We have accomplished this work in close association with members of the chronic fatigue syndrome self-help group, as many of the agencies we interviewed were suggested to us by contacts within the self-help community. As a result, many individuals with chronic fatigue syndrome from across the country have contacted our research team about setting up a housing program, and they have discussed their own difficulties in obtaining housing. A woman in California was forced to live in her van until she found housing. In addition, a man from Pennsylvania is beginning to set up congregate housing for people with chronic fatigue syndrome who might benefit from living in a toxic-free environment. We have shared this information with others across the country who are interested in establishing housing programs.

We also shared our findings on possible housing initiatives with members of the Chicago Chronic Fatigue Syndrome Association. Many thought that the programs described above could provide an important service to the people with chronic fatigue syndrome community. For one year, the university group collaborated with members of the Chicago Chronic Fatigue Syndrome Association in preparing a grant proposal to develop these types of housing initiatives. We are currently in the process of meeting with several foundations about this proposal.

We believe that the best way to start and maintain a viable housing program is to work collaboratively with those in need of housing. We began our work in this area by learning from organizations that already provided housing, even if the interventions had been developed for different populations. In this manner, we could provide people with chronic fatigue syndrome examples of successful programs and empower them to create and maintain similar programs. Collaboration between community psychologists and people with chronic fatigue syndrome allows both groups to work from a "strengths" perspective–with each group gaining insights and knowledge from the other. Thus by listening to the needs of each group and respectively involving each party in the decision making, each of the parties begins to trust the other, communications are facilitated and both parties can become more invested in, and committed to, the research process.

The ecological-collaborative model provided our group with the underlying theoretical model for working on this project. By bringing together self-help group members and students from university based settings, we believe that better social and community interventions, such as housing initiatives, can be developed that will allow us to more sensitively extend services to patients with chronic fatigue syndrome. The dearth of programs developed to date might be due to the fact that many physicians continue to believe that chronic fatigue syndrome is a psychiatric rather than a medical disorder. In such a situation, community psychologists can participate in assembling collaborative teams to develop service programs that are requested, but currently not available, to most people with this syndrome. These types of actions can allow community psychologists to help set the agenda for how service delivery programs are developed for people with chronic fatigue syndrome, and such activities could have influential roles in helping shape public policy.

DAILY ASSISTANCE

Another way in which community psychologists can intervene to empower persons with chronic fatigue syndrome, as well as individuals with other disabilities, is by developing volunteer caregiving programs. With people with chronic fatigue syndrome, helping with daily chores on a regular basis was perceived as one of the higher priority needs by the national sample (Jason et al., 1996).

In our first collaborative effort with the Chicago Chronic Fatigue Syndrome Association, Shlaes and Jason (1996) developed a program where people with chronic fatigue syndrome received a volunteer buddy and a mentor who had chronic fatigue syndrome. The buddy was an individual in the community who agreed to spend one hour a week conducting home visits with an individual with chronic fatigue syndrome. Buddy-participant matches were made based upon needs/ interests assessments completed by the participants and buddies. Mentors were individuals with chronic fatigue syndrome who were willing and able to engage in 2 hours of phone contact each month with the participants. The role of mentor was designed to include informational and emotional support. After the end of the program, the Chicago Chronic Fatigue Syndrome Association took over the mentorship portion of the program, and currently provides mentors to its members.

Our research team continues to work on developing and evaluating pilot volunteer programs for people with chronic fatigue syndrome. We are currently developing feedback systems to help people with chronic fatigue syndrome track their fatigue levels, energy and activities. One of the research forms we are using was devised by a member of the Chicago Chronic Fatigue Syndrome Association. Our research team had developed a global measure of expended energy on a daily basis. A member of the self-help group felt that a more precise instrument would better capture activities, so she developed this form and collected pilot data on the new instrument.

Much of the controversy surrounding illness management for chronic fatigue syndrome centers on the uncertainty regarding an appropriate balance between rest and activity. What has been slowly emerging from this debate is the prescription of energy conservation and the use of moderation (King, Jason, Frankenberry, Jordan, & Tryon, 1997). In our work with the volunteer program, we have learned that by avoiding overexertion, persons with chronic fatigue syndrome can avoid setbacks and relapses, while increasing their tolerance to activity. We believe suggestions for treatment plans and illness management need to be based upon individualized assessments and tailored to the patient's situation. For example, patients with chronic fatigue syndrome identified as continually overexerting themselves are advised to cut back and conserve their energy resources so that long-term gains in their tolerance to activity can be made. Our work suggests that all persons with chronic fatigue syndrome should not necessarily either increase or decrease their activity levels, instead what is needed is the use of moderation and energy conservation. This strategy, which we call the "envelope theory," was suggested to us by a member of the self-help program who had been provided a buddy.

Evidence exists that supports the energy conservation model described above. For example, in the Shlaes and Jason (1996) intervention study, participants who received the Buddy/Mentor intervention, and thus were able to conserve energy, experienced significant decreases in fatigue severity, while the control group experienced significant increases in fatigue severity. In addition, a time series study by Jason, King, Frankenberry, Jordan, and Tryon (1999) found that energy expended, physical exertion, and mental exertion were positively related to fatigue.

Not only do people with chronic fatigue syndrome benefit from having helpers, but volunteers benefit from their experience as well. Ferrari and Jason (1996) found that caregivers to people with chronic fatigue syndrome consistently reported more satisfaction than stress from care giving. This finding suggests that caregiving, in and of itself, can be a fulfilling experience that satisfies personal and emotional needs for the caregiver. By working directly with people with chronic fatigue syndrome, volunteers can learn a great deal about the lives of people with disabilities and the obstacles they need to overcome.

The program developed by Shlaes and Jason (1996) was our first mentor/buddy program, and we have continued to refine and develop our programming, with close input from the Chicago Chronic Fatigue Syndrome Association. Once again, an ecological model has guided our work on this project. At the present time, we have a joint committee of university researchers and self-help group members from the Chicago Chronic Fatigue Syndrome Association. The university personnel are recruiting volunteers for an expanded buddy program, and the members of the joint committee are involved in establishing a training program for volunteers and a system for jointly supervising the volunteers. In this way, both parties will be involved in all decision-making processes, and we expect both groups will be highly committed to these interventions.

OTHER COLLABORATIVE PROJECTS WITH THE CHICAGO CHRONIC FATIGUE SYNDROME ASSOCIATION

Our university volunteers have also assisted the Chicago Chronic Fatigue Syndrome Association in other capacities. For example, one research assistant helped the chronic fatigue syndrome group leader create a directory of resources for people with chronic fatigue syndrome in the Chicago metropolitan area. This resource directory has become an important asset to the organization, and its sales generate income for the self-help organization. The directory is now revised and updated each year by members of the self-help group. Members of our research teams have also assisted the chronic fatigue syndrome group leader with the assembling and mailing of the organization's newsletter, as well as the reorganization of their filing system. The help of healthy volunteers in these types of activities has been well received by the members of the chronic fatigue syndrome self-help group; it increases their commitment to our collaborative relationship.

Members from the CFS research team have also collaborated with the Chicago Chronic Fatigue Syndrome Association in an effort to assist children and parents of children who are suffering from CFS. To assess the needs of these children and their parents, our research team developed, in collaboration with members of the Chicago Chronic Fatigue Syndrome Association, a short survey of open- and closed-ended questions designed to evaluate the need for possible services. All of the mothers enthusiastically responded to the suggestion of organizing a support group so that their children could meet other children who are suffering from the CFS illness. This information was passed to the Executive Director of the Chicago Chronic Fatigue Association, who is currently working to serve the needs of these people.

DISCUSSION

Beginning in 1991, we began assembling a research team to work with individuals with chronic fatigue syndrome. At the time, there were few social services available for people with this illness. Our first priority was to collect data on the epidemiology of this syndrome. We felt that the most important need was to provide accurate estimates of the prevalence of this syndrome. We next began a collaborative relationship with the Chicago Chronic Fatigue Syndrome Association, based on an ecological model. A series of social and community interventions have been mounted to address issues such as employment, shared housing, and daily assistance. Through the process of developing and implementing these intervention models, both our research team and members of committees from the local chronic fatigue syndrome support group have benefited.

Much of the focus of this paper has been on collaboration between a self-help organization and university collaborators. In some cases, the intervention led to research, as with the buddy/mentor study and our subsequent development of a model of energy conservation. The Chicago Chronic Fatigue Syndrome Association benefited from a series of innovative demonstration projects provided to their members. Some of the pilot projects were incorporated into regular programming–the Chicago Chronic Fatigue Syndrome self-help group currently uses the resource directory and the mentor system. An excellent working relationship with the self-help group organization means undergraduate and graduate students have no difficulty recruiting participants from members of the self-help group when they need to interview participants with CFS for honors projects or theses. The members of the self-help group also have been instrumental in identifying areas for us to investigate, as the idea for the buddy/mentor system came from one of the self-help group members.

Our university-based community psychology resources supported and strengthened the directions determined by the self-help group. For example, using the youthful energy of university students to help persons with chronic fatigue syndrome achieve their independent living goals without formal agency involvement is a great resource-need match. This kind of multi-intervention effort has much potential for formulating an integrative perspective for community psychologists working with chronic fatigue syndrome, persons with other disabilities and with other "people in trouble."

Some readers may wonder whether chronic fatigue syndrome is a potentially reversible disability, such as a medical disorder that will eventually be addressed by pharmacological intervention. If so, then some might argue that the involvement of the community psychologist may be phased out as medical progress is made. The prospect for identifying a single etiological agent is uncertain, but even if it were to be identified, as with HIV/AIDS, there still would be a need for the development of service programs for those with this illness. Alternatively, if chronic fatigue syndrome does not have a clear cut etiology but is rather a complex disorder involving genetic, constitutional, environmental, and psychological factors, then medication might be palliative but not curative, and the role of the community psychologist will probably be larger and more enduring, involving both advocacy and health promotion.

Approaches to treatment must be comprehensive, addressing a variety of care needs. For example, advocacy focused on securing appropriate medical treatment and on the allocation of government resources for treatment has been cited as a high-priority need for individuals with chronic fatigue syndrome. People with chronic fatigue syndrome may desire (and need) an advocacy program in which the general public and the medical community becomes better educated about the problems and difficulties associated with chronic fatigue syndrome. Some patients with chronic fatigue syndrome may need assistance from others in order to complete daily living tasks. Living arrangements that include "healthy" individuals may be needed by people with chronic fatigue syndrome, because weakness from this illness might prevent them from accomplishing necessary chores. Finally, a sense of community in which mutual social support is promoted may prevent isolation, depression, and preoccupation with the illness among patients with chronic fatigue syndrome. A key question here concerns the highest priority needs, especially from the perspective of the patient with chronic fatigue syndrome. Collaborative research, as has been described throughout this paper, can be a key tool for helping set this agenda and work in mutually rewarding ways with self-help organizations. In this way, the needs of both parties are met, and both learn from each other and become invested in the relationship and interventions. The conclusions we have made concerning the benefits of collaboration, using an ecological model, also apply to working with people with other types of disabilities (e.g., people with osteoporosis who are homebound; people with energy management issues like some with cerebral palsy; and people facing public and professional skepticism and antipathy such as people with AIDS). An increasing knowledge of the different psychological, social, community, and medical factors accounting for chronic illnesses might help the field of community psychology develop more sophisticated models and more effective interventions. In addition, we become a more caring and humane society when we work collaboratively with community groups in investing resources in the establishment of decent living conditions for all our citizens.

REFERENCES

Davis, T.H., Jason, L.A., & Banghart, M.A. (1998). The effect of housing on individuals with multiple chemical sensitivities. *Journal of Primary Prevention, 19,* 31-42.

Ferrari, J.R., & Jason, L.A. (1997). A study of long-term volunteer caregiving to persons with CFS: Perceived stress vs. Satisfaction. *Rehabilitation Counseling Bulletin, 40,* 240-250.

Friedberg, F., & Jason, L.A. (1998). *Understanding chronic fatigue syndrome: An empirical guide to assessment and treatment.* Washington, D.C.: American Psychological Association.

Gunn, W.J., Connell, D.B., & Randall, B. (1993). Epidemiology of chronic fatigue syndrome: The Centers-for-Disease-Control study. In B.R. Bock & J. Whelan (Eds.), *Chronic Fatigue Syndrome.* (pp. 83-101). New York: John Wiley & Sons.

Jason, L.A., Ferrari, J.R., Taylor, R.R., Slavich, S.P., & Stenzel, C.L. (1996). A national assessment of the service, support, and housing preferences by persons with chronic fatigue syndrome: Toward a comprehensive rehabilitation program. *Evaluation and the Health Professions, 19,* 194-207.

Jason, L.A., King, C.P., Frankenberry, E.L., Jordan, K.M., Tryon, W.W., Rademaker, F., & Huang, C. (1999). Chronic fatigue syndrome: Assessing symptoms and activity level. *Journal of Clinical Psychology, 55,* 411-424.

Jason, L.A., Richman, J.A., Friedberg, F., Wagner, L., Taylor, R., & Jordan, K.M. (1997). Politics, science, and the emergence of a new disease: The case of Chronic Fatigue Syndrome. *American Psychologist, 52,* 973-983.

Jason, L.A., Taylor, R., Wagner, L., Holden, J., Ferrari, J.R., Plioplys, A. V., Plioplys, S., Lipkin, D., Papernik, M. (1995). Estimating rates of chronic fatigue syndrome from a community based sample: A pilot study. *American Journal of Community Psychology, 23,* 557-568.

Jason, L.A., Taylor, S.L., Johnson, S., Goldston, S., Salina, D., Bishop, P., & Wagner, L. (1993). Prevalence of Chronic Fatigue Syndrome-related symptoms among nurses. *Evaluation and the Health Professions, 16*(14), 385-399.

Jason, L. A., Wagner, L., Taylor, R., Ropacki, M.T., Shlaes, J., Ferrari, J., Slavich, S. P., & Stenzel, C. (1995). Chronic fatigue syndrome: A new challenge for health care professionals. *Journal of Community Psychology, 23,* 143-164.

Kelly, J.G. (1986). Context and process: An ecological view of the interdependence of practice and research. *American Journal of Community Psychology, 14,* 581-594.

King, C.P., Jason, L.A., Frankenberry, E.L., Jordan, K.M., & Tryon, W. (1997). Managing chronic fatigue syndrome through behavioral monitoring of energy levels and fatigue: A case study demonstration of the envelope theory. *The CFIDS Chronicle, 10,* 10-14.

Kingry-Westergaard, C., & Kelly, J.G. (1990). A contextualist epistemology for ecological research. In P. Tolan, C. Keys, F. Chertok, & L. Jason (Eds.) *Researching community psychology. Issues of theory and methods.* (pp. 23-31). Washington, DC.: American Psychological Association.

LeRoy, J., Davis, T.H., & Jason, L.A. (1996). Treatment efficacy: A survey of 305 MCS patients. *The CFIDS Chronicle, 9,* 52-53.

Maton, K.I. (1989). Towards an ecological understanding of mutual-help groups: The social ecology of "fit." *American Journal of Community Psychology, 17,* 729-753.

Serrano-Garcia, I. (1990). Implementing research: Putting our values to work. In P. Tolan, C. Keys, F. Chertok, & L. Jason (Eds.), *Researching community psychology: Issues of theory and methods* (pp.171-182). Washington, D.C.: American Psychological Association.

Shlaes, J.L., & Jason, L.A. (1996). A buddy/mentor program for people with chronic fatigue syndromes. *The CFIDS Chronicle, 9,* 21-25.

Vercoulen, J.H.M.M., Swanink, C.M.A., Fennis, J.F.M., Galama, J.M.D., van der Meer, J.W.M., & Bleijenberg, G. (1996), Prognosis in chronic fatigue syndrome: A prospective study on the natural course. *Journal of Neurology, Neurosurgery, and Psychiatry, 60,* 489-494.

Ware, N.C., & Kleinman, A. (1992). Culture and somatic experience: The social course of illness in Neurasthenia and Chronic Fatigue Syndrome. *Psychosomatic Medicine, 54,* 546-560.

Wilson, A., Hickie, I., Lloyd, A., Hadzi-Pavlovic, D., Boughton, C., Dwyer, J., & Wakefield, D. (1994). Longitudinal study of outcome of chronic fatigue syndrome. *British Medical Journal, 308,* 756-759.

Empowering Latinos with Disabilities to Address Issues of Independent Living and Disability Rights: A Capacity-Building Approach

Fabricio E. Balcazar
Christopher B. Keys

University of Illinois at Chicago

Yolanda Suarez-Balcazar

Loyola University of Chicago

SUMMARY. Latinos with disabilities have historically been underrepresented in efforts to set the disability agenda and promote disability rights. This manuscript describes a capacity-building approach to community empowerment. Our goal was to empower Latinos with disabilities, increasing their degree of control over services and decisions that directly affect them. The capacity-building approach is grounded in a

Address correspondence to: Dr. Fabricio Balcazar, Department of Disability and Human Development, University of Illinois at Chicago, 1640 West Roosevelt Road, Chicago, IL 60608.

This manuscript was funded in part by a grant from the National Institute on Disability and Rehabilitation Research (NIDRR), award number H133A40032 and by the Department of Disability and Human Development at the University of Illinois at Chicago.

[Haworth co-indexing entry note]: "Empowering Latinos with Disabilities to Address Issues of Independent Living and Disability Rights: A Capacity-Building Approach." Balcazar, Fabricio E., Christopher B. Keys, and Yolanda Suarez-Balcazar. Co-published simultaneously in *Journal of Prevention & Intervention in the Community* (The Haworth Press, Inc.) Vol. 21, No. 2, 2001, pp. 53-70; and: *People with Disabilities: Empowerment* and *Community Action* (ed: Christopher B. Keys, and Peter W. Dowrick) The Haworth Press, Inc., 2001, pp. 53-70. Single or multiple copies of this article are available for a fee from The Haworth Document Delivery Service [1-800-342-9678, 9:00 a.m. - 5:00 p.m. (EST). E-mail address: getinfo@haworth pressinc.com].

53

contextual/behavioral model of empowerment of people with disabilities. This approach emphasizes developing partnerships with local advocacy organizations and encourages active participation of people with disabilities and their families in identifying and addressing their own needs. Such capacity-building includes six major steps: (1) community entry and project planning; (2) identifying community concerns and strengths; (3) community organizing; (4) action planning; (5) monitoring and feedback; and (6) sustaining community organizing efforts. We illustrate the process with an example of an effort to promote compliance with the American with Disabilities Act in the Latino communities of Chicago, which resulted in over 70 actions and 24 outcomes over a period of 10 to 16 months. The capacity-building approach represents a community psychology effort to support ethnic minority individuals with disabilities in their struggle for equality and justice. To date, it has yielded encouraging results. Challenges for implementing this approach to community empowerment are discussed. *[Article copies available for a fee from The Haworth Document Delivery Service: 1-800-342-9678. E-mail address: <getinfo@haworthpressinc.com> Website: <http://www.Haworth Press.com> © 2001 by The Haworth Press, Inc. All rights reserved.]*

KEYWORDS. Capacity building, empowerment, coalition, Americans with Disabilities Act (ADA), physical disabilities, advocacy, Latinos(as)

The process of empowering community members to pursue their own agenda and address their needs has a long tradition in community psychology (Berger & Neuhaus, 1977; Rappaport, 1981; Rappaport & Seidman, in press). Empowerment refers to both individual determination over one's own life and democratic participation in one's community (Rappaport, 1987). Community empowerment in this case refers to the efforts of individuals with common concerns and characteristics to increase the degree of control over their own destiny and their capacity to influence bodies that make decisions that affect their community and its members. Despite the popularity of the concept of empowerment, there is still little agreement about the best strategies to actually increase the power of disenfranchised individuals (Rappaport & Seidman, in press). Previous models (e.g., Raeburn & Seymour, 1979; Raeburn, 1986) have proposed the utilization of needs assessment, goal setting, resource utilization, action, and feedback in the creation or improvement of community programs and services. This manuscript describes a community empowerment approach that first focuses on developing awareness and connections among various constituencies and then encourages and supports community change over time. Most of this research was derived from efforts to promote independent living goals among people with physical disabilities (Balcazar, Mathews, Francisco, Fawcett, & Seekins, 1994; Fawcett et al., 1994).

The proposed approach was developed in the context of the efforts of a local coalition of Latinos with disabilities and family members to improve compliance with the Americans with Disabilities Act (ADA) of 1990. The ADA is the most comprehensive civil rights law for individuals with disabilities to date. Modeled after the Civil Rights Act of 1964 and the Rehabilitation Act of 1973, the ADA is expected to have a significant impact on the working and living environments of citizens with disabilities. The law seeks to prohibit employer discrimination, remove transportation and communication barriers, and improve access to public goods and services (Johnson & Baldwin, 1993).

Many individuals are required to comply with the ADA, including employers, state and local government policy makers, business owners, and providers of goods and services. Under the act, they may have to remove architectural, communication, and accessibility barriers; modify rules, policies, and procedures; and provide auxiliary aids and services. Success of the ADA is highly dependent on the actions of those individuals, while enforcement and compliance promotion is in the hands of individuals with disabilities and their supporters.

On October 21, 1992, in San Francisco, California, the National Council on Disability held a public hearing on how minorities with disabilities are faring under the ADA. A major conclusion of this hearing was that "some minority groups like African and Native Americans with disabilities are over represented in the disability community, and that all minority groups are significantly under reached by current ADA information and technical assistance efforts" (Wright & Leung, 1993, p. 7). The individuals who testified at the ADA hearing on minority issues discussed their experiences with discrimination on the basis of disability and minority status, as well as their difficulty in gaining access to the resources needed to become self-sufficient. Minorities with disabilities often experience discrimination both on the basis of their culture and on the basis of their disability (Alston, Russo, & Miles, 1994). They have greater difficulty obtaining employment and gaining access to public accommodations and transportation than do whites with disabilities (Wright & Leung, 1993). Many Latinos with disabilities also have language and communication barriers that may complicate their ability to obtain meaningful information and technical assistance from local service agencies, including agencies whose mission consists of advocating and supporting persons with disabilities, such as Centers for Independent Living (CILs). They also have differences in cultural values and often share a sense of distrust of government policies and programs (Wright & Leung, 1993). Preliminary results from a process to identify the needs of Latinos with disabilities from the Chicago area, revealed that over 93% of respondents were not aware of their ADA rights and responsibilities (Balcazar & Keys, 1996).

Given that laws like the ADA require consumers and/or advocates to file formal complaints to seek improved compliance, efforts to promote awareness and advocacy among minority community members are urgently needed. Similar advocacy is needed by parents of children in special education, who often have to face hostile "Individual Educational Planning" committees and need to advocate for services for their children under the Individuals with Disabilities Education Act (IDEA). All these facts suggest the critical importance of developing the capacity of minority individuals with disabilities and their family members to take an active role in promoting awareness of and compliance with disability rights laws like the ADA and IDEA. The following is a description of the steps in the community capacity-building approach.

A CAPACITY-BUILDING APPROACH TO COMMUNITY EMPOWERMENT

This capacity-building approach was drawn from a decade of experiences in our Advocacy and Organizational Development Group at the Department of Disability and Human Development in the areas of self-advocacy and community empowerment, working in collaboration with people with all types of disabilities (Balcazar et al., 1994; Balcazar, Seekins, Fawcett, & Hopkins, 1990; Balcazar, Keys, & Garate-Serafini, 1995; Bartunek, Foster-Fishman, & Keys, 1996; Bond & Keys, 1993; Miller & Keys, 1996). This approach has been used effectively to affect decisions about programs, policies, budget allocations, and accessibility modifications in many communities (Balcazar et al., 1990; Balcazar et al., 1994).

Community capacity-building is a process by which individuals who share a common predicament can help and support each other, both in their efforts to pursue individual needs and in their efforts to develop a local agenda to address commonly identified needs. This process implies first the implementation of participatory strategies to identify community needs (e.g., Suarez-Balcazar, Bradford, & Fawcett, 1988), followed by the development of leaders and advocates who can plan and take action to address identified needs (e.g., Balcazar et al., 1994). This approach energizes the various constituency groups in the community and increases their level of communication, thereby facilitating mutual understanding. A capacity-building approach assumes that those individuals who are most negatively affected by current conditions–when given support and opportunities to make changes–are most likely to be committed and follow through with action. The approach first intends to promote synergy in the community as a result of the collaborative interaction between various constituency groups (e.g., individuals with various disabilities, their family members, and social agency personnel), who do not often work together (cf. Bartunek et al., 1996; Bond & Keys, 1993); once a local coalition is organized and a vision for the future of the community formulated, the emphasis turns to developing and implementing actions that address commonly identified needs and to sustaining those efforts over time.

The proposed approach to community empowerment has six phases, which are summarized in Table 1. In describing each phase, we will briefly identify its conceptual basis and components, discuss some potential limitations to implementation, possible solutions, and offer relevant examples. The illustrative examples are drawn from a recent application of this process with Latinos with disabilities and family members who participated in a project to promote compliance and awareness with the Americans with Disabilities Act (ADA) in the Chicago area. The community organizing effort can be started by a small group of individuals–*change agents*–and eventually be expanded to include many individuals and organizations. The change agents take the initial steps to organize the community coalition and promote the involvement of others in the process. They might include staff from a local agency, individuals with disabilities, researchers from a local college or university, or representatives from a state or national organization. We will now discuss each phase of the model.

TABLE 1. A Capacity-Building Approach to Community Empowerment

Phase I: COMMUNITY ENTRY AND PROJECT PLANNING

1. Contact local community agencies and advocacy groups
2. Identify potential leaders
3. Discuss project goals with potential leaders
4. Develop a strategy for funding the organizing effort (agency sponsorship, foundations, etc.)
5. Learn about the target community and its members
6. Recruit and train initial Coalition Group Members

Phase II: IDENTIFYING COMMUNITY STRENGTHS AND CONCERNS

1. Conduct focus groups to identify general needs and recruit volunteers to develop needs assessment survey
2. Conduct meeting to develop survey items
3. Prepare survey for distribution
4. Administer and collect needs assessment data
5. Analyze survey results and prepare list of community strengths and problems
6. Publicize findings of the needs assessment

Phase III: COMMUNITY ORGANIZING

1. Conduct public meeting to review identified problems
2. Discuss concerns and potential solutions
3. Specify coalition goals
4. Recruit volunteers for action groups
5. Help volunteers identify leaders and priorities for their action groups
6. Schedule regular meetings

Phase IV: PLANNING AND TAKING ACTION

1. Provide training to group leaders on how to run action-oriented meetings
2. Support action groups in planning and organizing activities
3. Support action groups in identifying local resources
4. Provide advocacy training to action group members as needed

Phase V: MONITORING/FEEDBACK

1. Collect copies of action planning logs from action groups
2. Provide feedback to group members about their action plans
3. Provide support to groups on their progress toward reaching goals
4. Celebrate goal attainment
5. Support action groups in the process of identifying new goals and targets for action

Phase VI: SUSTAINING COMMUNITY ORGANIZING EFFORTS

1. Develop new leaders and members
2. Reorganize around new members primary concerns
3. Support group efforts to secure resources for continuing operations

1. *Community Entry and Project Planning.* This initial phase involves developing a working relationship with community members and organizations. The entry process is multifaceted and continues throughout the life of the capacity-building effort as new organizations and individuals become involved in the process of community empowerment. Community entry is important at the outset to establish a basis for collaboration in project planning and in building trust between the community members and the researchers (Suarez-Balcazar, Balcazar, & Fawcett, 1992). The entry process requires the identification of key individuals and relevant organizations that participate and serve the target minority community. Organizations not only include those that specifically provide disability-related services, but also churches, schools, and social and political organizations. In addition, it is important to secure the cooperation of one or more established advocacy groups, as well as individuals in the community that include members of the minority group that will become involved in the capacity-building process. Potential barriers to effective community entry include relevant identity differences between the researchers and community members (e.g., race, class, disability, and/or gender), perceived and actual power differences (e.g., previous negative history of community members with university researchers), lack of preexisting community ties (e.g., the researcher is unknown to community members), and an overly directive approach to working with community members (e.g., a researcher who demands collaboration).

Change agents multiply their chances of developing broad support for their organizing efforts by cooperating with diverse local groups and organizations with direct ties to community members (Alinsky, 1946). After identifying potential leaders, change agents can learn more about the target community and the characteristics of its members through informal conversations with local leaders and other community members. Once a relationship develops, meetings of potential collaborators are organized to discuss disability issues in the community, articulate a vision for the future of the community, formulate initial project goals, and review the capacity-building approach. Such a participatory, collaborative approach to community entry can help overcome the barriers noted above.

In Chicago, we developed a grant proposal in collaboration with a local advocacy organization for Latinos with disabilities which was funded to implement the capacity-building process. We invited leaders and representatives from multiple organizations to a kick-off reception to promote and celebrate the start of the organizing effort. We later had a series of planning sessions with a group of local leaders in which all the components and steps of the capacity-building process were discussed. An implementation plan was developed and different individuals were assigned responsibilities for carrying out various tasks. Local leaders were invited to participate in the coalition–which we called the ADA Leadership Committee–and they in turn helped recruit additional volunteers for the needs assessment and action groups. These leaders also supported planning and organizing efforts in the community. Project staff included Latinos(as) with and without disabilities, some of whom were from the community.

2. *Identify Community Strengths and Concerns.* The needs assessment phase determines the direction of the organizing efforts and helps set the priorities for action in the community empowerment process. The capacity-building approach uses a modified version of a needs assessment and agenda setting methodology called the *concerns report method* (Fawcett, Suarez, Johnson, Whang-Ramos, Seekins, & Bradford, 1987; Fawcett, Seekins, Wang-Ramos, Muiu, & Suarez-Balcazar, 1984; Suarez-Balcazar, Bradford & Fawcett, 1988). This method systematically identifies community strengths and concerns from the perspective of individuals with disabilities and their family members. The concerns report method has been applied in over 350 communities and with the participation of more than 15,000 individuals with disabilities (Suarez-Balcazar et al., 1988).

Potential barriers to an effective needs assessment process include limited access to a representative sample of the target population; the cost associated in reproducing, distributing, and collecting surveys; potential lack of expertise in data analysis and reporting; and poor community participation in the town meetings. Appropriate planning, networking, and advertising of the needs assessment process can alleviate most of these problems.

In Chicago, the first step in the needs assessment process was to work with a community partner agency–an advocacy organization for Latinos with disabilities–to organize three focus groups with target consumers and family members in order to identify ADA-related needs of Latinos in the community. We then recruited from those groups a representative group of about 10 individuals who developed a brief survey based on the information collected from the focus groups. The survey had approximately 20 questions addressing key areas of accessibility to employment, goods and services, local and federal services, and telecommunications. The survey had two types of questions for each item: one question asked about the *importance* of the particular issue (from 1 'not important' to 4 'very important'); the other, about the individual's *satisfaction* with the community's effort to address the issue (from 1 'not satisfied' to 4 'very satisfied'). This format allows the identification of both community strengths (i.e., items rated with high importance and satisfaction scores) and community concerns (i.e., items with high importance and low satisfaction scores) (Fawcett et al., 1987).

The questionnaire was developed in English and translated into Spanish using standard double translation techniques (i.e., translated from English to Spanish and then from Spanish to English to verify accuracy) (Brislin, 1986). The Spanish version was reviewed by community leaders and coalition members. To review different options for survey distribution, see Fawcett et al. (1982). We used small group administration of the survey as a culturally sensitive mode of data collection to provide support to respondents and answer questions. We collected approximately 60 surveys in 5 sessions. In some cases, it was necessary to make adaptations for people with special needs, such as providing a large print or a taped copy for individuals with visual disabilities (see Suarez-Balcazar, Balcazar, & Keys, 1997 for additional survey instructions).

3. *Community Organizing.* This phase focuses on recruiting the individuals who are going to take the actions in the community empowerment effort. Once the results of the needs assessment surveys are identified, public forums are held to: (a) inform people with disabilities and their families of the disability-related issues and concerns identified by community members; (b) increase their awareness about disability issues in general; (c) provide participants with an opportunity to brainstorm solutions to the issues identified; and (d) become part of action committees to work on the issues of most concern to those attending the forum. The last process becomes the community organizing effort by involving participants in *action groups*. The change agents organizing the forum at this time help group members specify goals and continue to recruit volunteers for the action groups. The change agents support the action groups and assist group members in identifying facilitators for each group. When the members of the

group get together for the first time, they select a convenient time to continue meeting on a regular basis.

Potential barriers to community organizing include insufficient interest or awareness in the community about the organizing effort; little interest among town meeting participants in signing up to join action groups; and lack of volunteers to lead the action groups. An active participatory process of needs assessment, phone calls to potential participants, mailings, and posted fliers usually generate substantial interest in the forum. Providing opportunities for community members to discuss issues of concern in small groups is typically effective in engaging participants so that they want to join action groups.

In Chicago, during the public forum on ADA-related issues, which was attended by approximately 60 community members, participants were asked to specify how the issues identified affected them. Participants were also invited to discuss alternatives for addressing four of the main problems identified–problems with public transportation, lack of employment opportunities for people with disabilities, inappropriate services for children with disabilities in special education classrooms, and lack of awareness about the ADA in the Latino community. Forum participants were asked to meet in small groups to talk about the problem that most interested them. Committee members discussed the dimensions of the issues and brainstormed potential solutions thereby initiating the community empowerment process. In order to lead consumers into more sustained involvement, the small group discussion leaders recruited volunteers to participate in ongoing action groups.

4. *Planning and Taking Actions.* Action groups are one way in which people who share a common concern can work together toward a specific goal designed to improve the overall quality of life for people with disabilities and their families. Action groups seem to work best when members are consistently taking concrete actions on particular issues of importance to them both in and out of meetings. We encourage group leaders to attend regular monthly planning meetings to review action plans, share progress toward objectives, and provide feedback to each other. We also advise group members to use action logs in order to keep track of their actions and accomplishments (e.g., what is the objective of the action, actions needed to accomplish each objective, who is responsible for doing what and when?). A common problem in many consumer advocacy groups is the disorganization of

the leaders, lack of appropriate planning, and uneven participation of group members in the action process. Poor attendance at action group meetings can also become a problem. Strategies to reinforce group attendance include making clear progress on relevant issues, offering food or snacks during meetings, providing free baby sitting services, and car pooling. Initially, pairing community members with change agents for group leadership can make it easier for members to volunteer for leadership positions and can help make meetings more effective. In addition, training group participants increases relevant knowledge, improves advocacy skills, and helps group leaders in conducting effective meetings. Change agents can be instrumental in offering opportunities for group members to network and connect with other groups and organizations at the local, state, and even national levels.

In Chicago, the purpose of the ADA action committees was to facilitate the organizing of community members around ADA-related issues on which they wanted to take action. Committee members chose a convenient place and time to meet (e.g., second Saturday mornings of each month at a local library). We also had one staff member from the project supporting each committee and others providing child care, refreshments and transportation. Group leaders received training on how to run action-oriented meetings (Balcazar, Seekins, & Fawcett, 1994). During this phase, group members met regularly to identify and discuss solutions to identified issues. Training manuals are available from the authors upon request. Some individual participants have moved on to occupy community leadership positions in their local school councils; on agency boards; and civic organizations. Group members also organized an ADA campaign on disability rights with the local Spanish-speaking TV stations using public service announcements obtained from the New Jersey ADA Disability and Business Technical Assistance Center.

5. *Monitoring/Feedback.* Consistent with empowerment principles, action group members themselves select priorities and develop the action strategies to address identified needs (Miller & Keys, 1996). Consumers decide which issues to target for action. We encourage change agents to collect records of groups' progress and to feed back the information to the coalition members so they can appreciate and celebrate their progress. This step is important to reinforce people's sense of effectiveness and empowerment and to assess the overall progress of the community capacity-building effort. The data may

suggest the need for providing additional support and training to leaders and action group members. It may also suggest the need to redirect efforts or to encourage leaders to pursue new issues. The feedback process allows members of the coalition to estimate their progress in addressing community needs, the directions that consumers are taking in the process, and their relative effectiveness. Some groups might need assistance on how to make progress on specific issues. It is also possible that some groups may encounter very stern opposition or that group members choose direct confrontation tactics to address an issue. It helps to have some experienced advocates available for consultation as needed. It is also important that participants are fully aware of the potential risks of advocacy. An advocacy action-planning guide (Seekins, Balcazar, & Fawcett, 1986) was developed to help participants make informed decisions when planning an advocacy campaign. Finally, the information that the coalition collects from group leaders can also be used to publicize the community organizing efforts in the local media. Newspaper reports, TV and radio interviews can increase community support and encourage more people with disabilities to get involved.

In Chicago, we asked each group leader to prepare a monthly report of group actions to be shared with the members of the coalition. Coalition members provided verbal and/or written comments and suggestions about a particular action. Figure 1 displays the cumulative number of actions reported by members of the three ADA groups (employment, public accommodations, and special education services) for a period of 10 to 16 months. A total of 70 actions and 24 resulting outcomes were identified, including 14 community education events (e.g., presentations to local chambers of commerce); 5 fundraising events (e.g., chocolate bar sales); 3 changes in services (e.g., establishment of a new support group for visually impaired Latinos); 1 policy change in the eligibility criteria for a training program for parents in a local agency; and 1 board appointment to the Regional Transit Authority Advisory Board. This effort has continued and expanded beyond the period of the grant funding.

6. *Sustaining Community Organizing Efforts.* Two key steps for sustaining the capacity-building process include (1) ongoing member and leader development and (2) willingness to reorganize around new member concerns. We encourage members to provide additional leadership training for new leaders as needed. Recruiting new members for

FIGURE 1. The cumulative number of actions reported by the members of three community action groups: employment, special education services, and public accommodations. The arrows indicate times of meetings during which new goals were set.

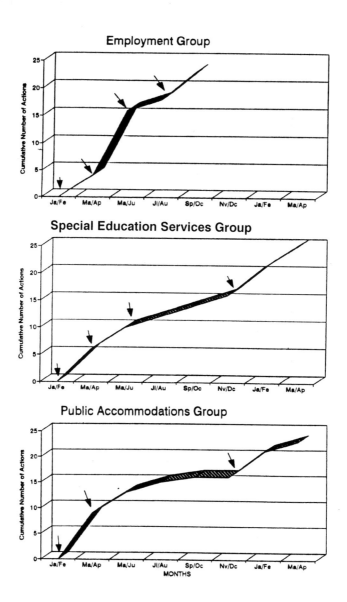

the action committees is essential for a sustained effort over time. Asking existing members to invite other people with disabilities and/ or their families to join is one way to sustain membership. To facilitate their entry into the group, new members are asked to start working on projects with more experienced consumers. Leaders can provide guidance and support to new group members, as well as giving them an overview of the process, a summary of previous accomplishments, and a detailed description of current projects. In some cases, training sessions can be organized to introduce new members to effective advocacy strategies and tactics. To keep participants involved and in contact with each other, we encourage leaders to call group members who are absent from meetings to find out how they are doing, to inform them of progress, and to include their views on group activities. Coalition members should also consider fund-raising activities to address short and long-term financial needs.

In Chicago, the arranging of the action groups around ADA issues like employment and accessibility did not always tap the central concern of the community participants. We have supported a restructuring of the action groups to focus on the perceived subgroups preferred by community participants. Several individual groups formed as a result of this capacity-building effort and are now providing needed services in the community (e.g., a group of parents of Latino children who are deaf; a group of Latinos who are visually impaired; and a group of mothers of Latino children attending special education classes). This new arrangement provided the incentive for them to continue their efforts into the future. We are currently assisting these new organizations to pursue local funding sources and they have already secured some logistical (e.g., meeting space) and technical support (e.g., how to file for tax exempt status) from local organizations.

CONCLUSION

We have presented an approach for building the capacity of community members to become empowered and increase their degree of control over relevant resources, services and opportunities. The process was illustrated with information from our experiences in building the capacity of Latinos with disabilities from the Chicago area. Community empowerment in this case involved multiple agents including university personnel, a community partner organization, community members, new community organizations and groups, and an organizing coalition working on commonly identified issues. As Miller and Keys (1996) and Zimmerman (in press) have noted, an empowerment approach redefines the professional's role as one of collaborator and facilitator rather than expert and counselor. We worked *with* the participants rather than advocating *for* them. We provided resources to the community, rather than imposing our values or perspectives. The process resulted in an increased level of involvement of Latinos with disabilities and family members in determining the services and decisions made to address their needs. Three new consumer-led organizations developed as a result of this process of transferring direct control and responsibility to the participants themselves.

We have successfully used this capacity-building approach to develop competencies and involve consumers in the decision-making process, empowering them to advance the agenda of Latinos with disabilities in the city. We are now working closely with a number of consumers and parents of children with disabilities who are involved in creating and running their own advocacy organizations. The capacity-building process had the beneficial effect of developing the leadership of individuals with disabilities and family members as advocates. In many cases, this advocacy process begins by encouraging people with disabilities to become active members of the community. Such attempts often reveal the types of barriers to community accessibility that individuals with disabilities confront. Effective advocacy can open up opportunities for individuals with disabilities to become employed and begin to address the biggest barrier of all–the pervasive poverty that affects so many people with disabilities.

The capacity-building process, however, is complex and potentially challenging. We pointed out several pitfalls of the process and steps that could be taken to overcome those limitations. The list of potential problems was not intended to be exhaustive, and future replications will add information about the limitations and benefits of this approach. Future replications may also identify contextual and individual strengths and barriers that affect community members as they seek to address their own needs. An important lesson learned from this experience is that the basic organizing units are not necessarily specific rights, but rather the common characteristics that people share. Although we started the action groups according to ADA issues and community members did take action to address ADA concerns (e.g., employment, public education, public transportation, and community awareness), participants subsequently organized themselves according to their personal interests. Although most participants shared issues like unemployment, or lack of accessibility for people with disabilities in the community, there were enough differences to justify this reorganization. Future organizing efforts would probably benefit by focusing the needs assessment process first on the specific needs of natural subgroups (e.g., parents of school age children with disabilities; various types of disabilities, etc.), and then on shared concerns. The individual groups can then advance their own projects, and the coalition can provide common ground for addressing shared concerns and continuing the coalition-building process. The coalition plays an important role in facilitating support among the leaders of the various organizations, and of providing the context for common advocacy efforts (e.g., a letter writing campaign to address state or federal changes in disability policy and services).

To conclude, from a conceptual point of view, we hope this work will expand the understanding of the process of community empowerment and of how communities can organize to address their own needs. The capacity-building approach to community empowerment led Latinos with disabilities and their families in Chicago to accomplish many relevant goals and to organize new consumer groups that continue to operate independently. They are now building coalitions and developing support networks that reflect their greater sense of confidence and a realization that united and organized they can succeed. As Rappaport (1987) said, "empowerment suggests a belief in the power of people to be both the masters of their own fate and involved in the life of their several communities" (p. 142). That is the path that Latinos with disabilities in the city of Chicago are building.

REFERENCES

Alinsky, S. (1946). *Reveille for radicals.* New York: Vintage Books.

Alston, R. J., Russo, C. J., & Miles, A. S. (1994). Brown vs Board of Education and the Americans with Disabilities Act: Vistas of equal educational opportunities for African Americans. *Journal of Negro Education, 63,* 349-357.

Balcazar, F. E., & Keys, C. B. (1996). *Developing the capacity of minority communities to address issues of independent living and disability rights.* Grant proposal, Institute on Disability and Human Development, Chicago, IL.

Balcazar, F. E., Keys, C. B., & Garate-Serafini, T. (1995). Learning to recruit assistance to attain transition goals: A program for adjudicated youth with disabilities. *Remedial and Special Education, 16,* 237-246.

Balcazar, F. E., Mathews, R. M., Francisco, V. T., Fawcett, S. B., & Seekins, T. (1994). The empowerment process in four advocacy organizations of people with disabilities. *Rehabilitation Psychology, 39(3),* 281-295.

Balcazar, F. E., Seekins, T., & Fawcett, S. B. (1994). *Consumer involvement in advocacy organizations: Changing communities for better living. Volume II: Conducting effective meetings.* Institute on Disability and Human Development, Chicago, IL.

Balcazar, F. E., Seekins, T. W., Fawcett, S. B., & Hopkins, B. L. (1990). Empowering people with physical disabilities through advocacy skills training. *American Journal of Community Psychology, 18,* 281-296.

Bartunek, J. M., Foster-Fishman, P. G., & Keys, C. B. (1996). Using collaborative advocacy to foster intergroup cooperation: A joint insider-outsider investigation. *Human Relations, 49,* 701-733.

Berger, P. L., & Neuhaus, R. J. (1977). *To empower people: The role of mediating structures in public policy.* Washington, D.C.: American Enterprise Institute for Public Policy Research.

Bond, M., & Keys, C. B. (1993). Empowerment, diversity, and collaboration: Promoting synergy on community boards. *American Journal of Community Psychology, 21,* 37-57.

Brislin, R. W. (1986). The wording and translation of research instruments. In R. W. Brislin (Ed.). *Field methods in cross-cultural research.* Beverly Hills, CA: Sage Publications (pp. 137-164).

Fawcett, S. B., Seekins, T., Whang-Ramos, P., Muiu, C., & Suarez-Balcazar, Y. (1982). Involving consumers in decision-making. *Social Policy, 13(6),* 36-41.

Fawcett, S. B., Suarez, Y., Johnson, M., Whang-Ramos, P., Seekins, T., & Bradford, B. (1987). *The disabled citizens concerns report manual.* Bureau of Child Research & the Research and Training Center on Independent Living, University of Kansas, Lawrence, KS.

Fawcett, S. B., White, G. W., Balcazar, F. E., Suarez-Balcazar, Y., Mathews, M. R., Paine-Andrews, A., Seekins, T., & Smith, J. F. (1994). A contextual-behavioral model of empowerment: Case studies involving people with physical disabilities. *American Journal of Community Psychology, 22,* 471-496.

Johnson, W. G., & Baldwin, M. (1993). The Americans with Disabilities Act: Will it make a difference? *Policy Studies Journal, 21,* 775-788.

Miller, A., & Keys, C. B. (1996). Awareness, action, and collaboration: How the self-advocacy movement is empowering for persons with developmental disabilities. *Mental Retardation, 34,* 312-319.

Rappaport, J. (1981). In praise of paradox: A social policy of empowerment over prevention. *American Journal of Community Psychology, 9,* 1-25.

Rappaport, J. (1987). Terms of empowerment/exemplars of prevention: Toward a theory for community psychology. *American Journal of Community Psychology, 15,* 121-145.

Rappaport, J., & Seidman, E. (2000). *Handbook of community psychology.* New York: Plenum Press.

Raeburn, J. M. (1986). Toward a sense of community: Comprehensive community projects and community houses. *Journal of Community Psychology, 14,* 391-398.

Raeburn, J. M., & Seymour, F. W. (1979). A simple systems model for community programs. *Journal of Community Psychology, 7,* 290-297.

Seekins, T., Balcazar, F. E., & Fawcett, S. B. (1986). *Consumer involvement in advocacy organizations.* Research and Training Center on Independent Living, University of Kansas, Lawrence, KS.

Suarez-Balcazar, Y., Balcazar, F. E., & Keys, C. B. (1997). *A self-help guide for community needs assessment and action planning.* Institute on Disability and Human development, University of Illinois at Chicago, Chicago, IL.

Suarez-Balcazar, Y., Balcazar, F. E., & Fawcett, S. B. (1992). Problem identification in social intervention research. In F. R. Bryant et al. (Eds.) *Methodological issues in applied social psychology.* New York: Plenum Press.

Suarez-Balcazar, Y., Bradford, B., & Fawcett, S. B. (1988). Common concerns of disabled Americans: Issues and options. *Social Policy, 19,* 29-35.

The *Americans with Disabilities Act of 1990.* Public Law 101-336, 42 U.S.C. & 12101 (1990).

Wright, T. J., & Leung, P. (1993). *Meeting the unique needs of minorities with disabilities: A report to the President and the Congress.* National Council on Disability, Washington, D.C.

Zimmerman, M. A. (2000). Empowerment theory: Psychological, organizational, and community levels of analysis. In J. Rappaport & E. Seidman (Eds.), *Handbook of Community Psychology.* New York: Plenum.

Community Responsiveness: Examples from Under-Resourced Urban Schools

Peter W. Dowrick

Center for Disability Studies (UAP) University of Hawaii

Thomas J. Power
Patricia H. Manz

Children's Seashore House and University of Pennsylvania

Marika Ginsburg-Block

University of Minnesota

Stephen S. Leff

Children's Seashore House and University of Pennsylvania

Soon Kim-Rupnow

Center for Disability Studies (UAP) University of Hawaii

SUMMARY. The ability of university-based programs to be responsive to the community takes more than good will and topical expertise. The needs

Address correspondence to: Professor Peter W. Dowrick, Center for Disability Studies, 1776 University Avenue, UA 4-6, University of Hawaii, Manoa, HI 96822 (E-mail: dowrick@hawaii.edu).

Portions of this paper have been presented at several national conferences, including the 14th Annual Pacific Rim Conference on Disabilities, Honolulu, February 1998. Activities were supported by the US Department of Education [H180G-70001], Pew Charitable Trusts, and the Annenberg Foundation, but the views expressed herein are solely those of the authors.

are more pressing than ever in urban schools in *low income* communities, where students with disabilities receive the least resources. This article describes a six-element approach of community responsiveness applied in the context of elementary schools in Pennsylvania, Hawaii, and beyond. These elements include: (1) community identification of its needs and strengths; (2) establishing a place in the system; (3) working as a resource; (4) building community capacity; (5) creating and using positive images; and (6) data-based, participatory evaluation. We illustrate this approach with the *ACE Reading* (literacy) and *PLAYS* (safe and productive recess) programs–addressing the two greatest concerns identified by our schools. These programs are fully inclusive of children with and without identified disabilities, and are designed to reduce the likelihood of special education classifications. These main outcomes indicate the potency of community capacity building on student, school, and systems development, using criterion-based monitoring and positive frameworks. The programs proved economical, costing in the vicinity of $10,000 per year (each school) to be implemented subsequently in 20 additional schools. The programs' descriptions and outcomes serve to illustrate a model of *community responsiveness. [Article copies available for a fee from The Haworth Document Delivery Service: 1-800-342-9678. E-mail address: <getinfo@haworthpressinc.com> Website: <http://www.HaworthPress.com> © 2001 by The Haworth Press, Inc. All rights reserved.]*

KEYWORDS. Urban schools, reading failure, low income communities, children with disabilities, community partners, social skills

Our work has increasingly focused on under-resourced communities, in common with other community scientists and activists; see Black and Krishnakumar, 1998; Schorr, 1997; Wilson, 1996; Zins, 1997. Since 1995, we have been working with schools in low income urban areas of large cities. In these areas, about 90% of children qualified for free or reduced lunch at school, 80% were African-American *or* immigrant (Samoan, Vietnamese, Filipino) families, they lived in the lowest 20% of housing amenities of their cities, and 50% of heads of households had graduated from high school (US Census, 1990). The communities' schools had high rates of dropout, and were in the bottom 30% for achievement in basic academics (Hawaii Department of Education, 1998; University of Pennsylvania Library, 1998; US Census, 1990). In such schools, half the children with "special education" classifications are designated because they are either two or more years behind academically or because of preventable challenging behaviors.

Such needs deserve best practices. How can exemplary services be implemented in those communities, and how can they be made to work? Not only are these questions driven by the needs of communities and their schools, there is the issue of "research to practice"–or more correctly "proven practice to adoption." That is, society needs effective and economic solutions, with sustainable implementation (Connell, Kubisch, Schorr, & Weiss, 1995). For example, reading specialists are trained to provide excellent support for students, but given the extent of the need described here, there are not enough of them and they cost too much. Likewise, there are social skills programs and trainers, too few and too costly for the needs (Chung & Elias, 1996; Anderson, 1993).

MODEL OF APPROACH

To respond to the situations indicated, we used a six-element approach of *community responsiveness* (Dowrick, 1998), supported by community psychology principles (Tolan, Keys, Chertok, & Jason, 1990). Designing effective intervention programs in urban community settings is a challenge requiring a balance between the need for methodological rigor to ensure the development of effective and replicable programs, and for procedural flexibility to be responsive to the needs and goals of the community. The following model was successfully used to develop intervention programs that were both community responsive and scientifically sound, regardless of individual disability labels, and often avoiding the need for them. See Table 1 for an overview. The *Specific Interventions* section later in this paper illustrates this model with examples from two programs.

1. Identification of Needs and Strengths of the Community by the Community

The intervention team collaborates with stakeholders in the community to identify the issues to be targeted for change, based on strengths as well as needs. Community members usually define the broad area in need of change, and experts assist in developing the specificity that can provide a basis for program development (Gresham & Lopez, 1996). For instance, community leaders might mention interracial tensions in the neighborhood and experts on the team could ask about incidents, locations, and broader events in the area. Community members provide a local cultural perspective and they can identify natural resources (e.g., church organizations) within their neighborhoods. Diversities, including 'disabilities,' usually create needs and strengths.

2. Establishing a Place in the System–By Informed Invitation

We never bring our 'models of change' or 'best practices' anywhere unless we are invited. That does not mean sitting in an office all day, waiting for the phone to ring. An invitation can be attained proactively. In areas in which we are already established, we have simply asked for support. A reputation is sometimes spread through newspapers or television–but more often by word of mouth or when a colleague moves to a new location. We may actively inform possible sites about program models and then respond to interest and invitation. In new areas, we might make a request for a meeting, sending a one page letter with a one page summary, or perhaps a news clipping of previous work. If new *and* without a track record, it pays to work with an insider, or at least to find some personal connection.

3. Working Relationship–A Resource to the Community

Relationships are established and developed on the community turf. Thus there are many issues of showing and gaining trust and respect, based on personnel, locations, and interactions (Manz, Power, Ginsburg-Block, & Dowrick, 1999). It is important, obviously, to include team members who are proactively responsive to the culture and competent, or capable of becoming competent, in it. It is essential to identify key people in the community and their roles. For instance, some schools are functionally run, day to day, by their secretaries. Training of

TABLE 1. Six Elements in the Model of Our Approach

Community Responsiveness
1. Identification of Needs and Strengths of the Community by the Community
2. Establishing a Place in the System–By Invitation
3. Working Relationship–A Resource to the Community
4. Capacity Building with Community Partners–Responsibility and Empowerment
5. Positive Visions, Creating Images of Future Success
6. Data-Based Evaluation, Participatory Action Research

project staff is best done in the location and situation in which it applies: if monitors are needed to prevent trouble during a cultural parade, they are better taught in the street during a similar event, than in the classroom. Therefore, the project needs an onsite location. Staff are taught how to interact with a broad range of circumstances that *may* arise–not just the ones they expect to be part of the job.

4. Capacity Building with Community Partners–Beyond Empowerment

The key principle is to empower as many individuals in the community as possible (Schorr, 1997). Tasks include identifying and recruiting community members, providing skills training, adding roles and responsibilities, supporting local values, language, and culture, giving everyone a voice, and improving communication (Manz et al., 1999). Children and adults can provide models, problem solving, and links to other community resources. Communities typically have a broad range of resources and multiple individuals who can serve as change agents. In schools, for example, parents can be trained to improve students' academic skills and school aides can be trained to improve social skills on the playground. Children themselves can be trained to use self-management or to provide support to their peers (Ginsburg-Block & Fantuzzo, 1998). Capacity building for local agents of change is doubly valuable for people with disabilities and other diversity.

5. Positive Visions–Creating Images of Future Success

Humans learn from observing success–including one's own success and images of success not yet achieved (Dowrick, 1999). The means include: goal setting, feedforward, fostering empowerment, increasing current opportunities for success, and positive relabeling. Appropriate goal setting is responsive to community perceptions of valuable outcomes and to expert opinion of meaningful change. As our community partners learn new roles, we support them with feedforward, not feedback (Dowrick, 1999). That is, we minimize attention to errors in past performance but rather celebrate current successes and describe potential futures–sometimes by creating video images of them. Community participants are recruited into coordinating and supervising roles as soon as feasible, first with sufficient support to maintain mastery, then with that support systematically withdrawn. We design instructional and social contexts to promote high rates of success. Failures are not punished but reframed as opportunities to learn, a favorable strategy for students with and without disabilities.

6. Data-Based Evaluation, Participatory Action Research

As many aspects of our interventions as possible are monitored, evaluated, and improved with objective and subjective data. Those who participate as 'subjects' also participate in the design, administration, and interpretation of the interventions (White, Nary, & Froelich, this volume; Whyte, 1991). Monitoring *integrity* and *performance* keeps the project and its interventions on track and enables ongoing improvements. We find written protocols, intervention checklists, observations, regular meetings, and other frequent listening interactions to be important. Non-critical feedback, based on time intervals (not on incidents), is also used. In our schools' programs, diverse educators, paraprofessionals, family members, students, and other community members (with and without disabilities) participate at every feasible level. Community partners monitor themselves and each other, collecting outcome data, and offering opinions on the assistive technology. They and the educators share in the decision making, the presentations, and the interpretation of the results.

SPECIFIC INTERVENTIONS: READING AND RECESS

The programs described here began in 1995, in the elementary schools of west and southwest urban Philadelphia. Some of these neighborhoods are 99% African-American; others are mixed with Caucasian, and Vietnamese and Cambodian immigrant families. In 1998, we expanded the program to urban Honolulu, to a community of mostly Samoan and Filipino cultures, with some Hawaiian and a sprinkling of half a dozen other ethnicities. We have since spread our efforts to other areas of Philadelphia (including Italian and Puerto Rican neighborhoods), to rural Hawaiian areas on different islands, including middle and high schools, and to the state of Kentucky. In response to different needs in these communities, our programs include childhood literacy, recess activities, structured lunchrooms, social skills, medical 'safety net,' transitions, recreation, local culture, science, homework, and the support of teachers regarding student conduct. Here we describe the literacy, *ACE Reading*, and recess, *PLAYS*, programs in three urban schools to illustrate our model of community responsiveness. ACE = Accelerated Community Empowerment; PLAYS = Playground, Lunchroom, And Youth Survival.

What our originating schools had in common was the lack of conventional resources to meet high levels of need. Most areas to which we have taken these programs also share this characteristic. The communities have more than 50% of families on welfare and many of the adults do not read or do not enjoy reading. The majority of children (50%-90%, varying across location and classroom) read below grade level. At the Honolulu school, 40% have English as their second language. The schools are all 'Title I,' that is, they qualify for federal assistance on the basis of the number of children (in our case, 80%) who qualify for free or reduced-cost breakfast and lunch. However, the schools remain under-resourced. Although they have libraries and sufficient teaching staff, they have minimal resources, such as budget, specialized personnel, and support staff to meet the extraordinary needs.

Identification of Needs and Strengths of the Community by the Community

Each of the schools in which we worked had experienced, established staff who were acutely aware of local needs through observations, staff and parent meetings, and through attempting to meet the standards expected by their districts. The schools also had a number (about 10 each) of local parents as employees or volunteers, some of whom were active in school administrative committees. We had several meetings with principals and other individuals to identify their perception of needs.

The primary concern initially expressed and echoed for 3 years was literacy: the large number of children not learning to read in the early grades and never catching up. A close second was concern for aggressive interactions, from overt violence to gossiping and excluding others during play. As well as spoiling the quality of school life, both these issues were identified by staff as contributing to the misidentification of students in later grades as "learning or behavior disabled." Other issues, addressed by us but not described here, included: access to services for student health and mental health and transitions of students both in and out of the catchment area and advancing to middle school, especially for students with special needs.

We were readily able to verify the levels of need by objective measures. The reading levels are noted above. Two of the schools retained one in five students for a second year in first grade–almost entirely based on reading proficiency. At one school we did a thorough screening of first grade students using a large (30%) random sample (Manz et al., 1999). The results showed that less than 5% of students were reading better than at a "frustrational" level on preprimer instructional materials.

To verify the needs in the playground environment, we scheduled a series of meetings with the principal, guidance counselor, physical education teacher, and playground assistants–who were parents and grandparents from the community, hired as paraprofessionals or volunteers. School staff and playground assistants expressed concern about physical aggression, teasing, and the lack of interaction among students of different ethnic groups. We also spoke to children who told us what they liked and did not like about recess. Through a series of observations, it became clear that playground supervision was rudimentary and inconsistent (Leff, Costigan, Ginsburg-Block, Rudnicki, & Power, 1998). For example, communication among supervisors was poor, students had equipment for very few games, and assistants often did not provide adequate coverage of the grounds.

A major strength was the community membership. Each school employed 10-15 local people as educational assistants, some with training in tutoring or recess supervision. Some had the respect of school educators and students. In all our neighborhoods, there were cultural strengths of caring about family and neighbors. The school personnel recognized these resources were underused.

Establishing a Place in the System–By Invitation

In our first school in this project, we were invited by the counselor because of the perceived needs she thought we and our colleagues might address. After establishing good faith (and good data) by our activities in the school, we were invited into another school in a nearby community. We then received some major federal funding to work in both the schools. In retrospect, we would have preferred to involve more school personnel and community members in the fundamentals of the funding proposal's conceptualization and development (cf. Chavis, Speer, Resnick, & Zippay, 1993). But tight timeframes compromised the quality of these communications. As we wrote other proposals and schools contracted with us using their own monies, we became able to gain earlier community participation–although school personnel continued to look to us to do most of the proposal work.

In all schools, we had strong support from the principal and the counselor. We were further assisted by the good fortune of public relations initiatives, resulting in a full range of media coverage: in-house news, syndicated newspapers, radio, television, and the world wide web. In Honolulu we identified potential sites and sent them a cover letter and newspaper article (Collins, 1997). Thus, a suitable urban school in this area adopted us and our reading program. Similar documents provided the foundation for partnerships in rural Hawaii, the state of Kentucky, and other locations.

However, the invitation by the school administrator is just the beginning. We had to earn our invitation on a recurring basis from teachers, assistants, and secretaries. We made presentations at staffings and identified key individuals (different at each school–receptionist, gym teacher, librarian) for additional conversations. We added staff members to our team who could represent a major cultural presence in each school–African-American, Vietnamese, Samoan. We emphasized the roles of tutors as mentors and recast the playground aides as "social skills trainers." The potential for self-determination was featured through the use of positive self-images, including video futures.

The Working Relationship–Resource to the Community

Once invited into a community, we consolidate by developing the working relationships–through personnel, locations, and interactions. Projects such as ours require operating locations–another scarce resource in these schools. As part of establishing an acceptable place in the system, we found ourselves painting a basement room at one school, sharing a trailer at another, and providing furniture and equipment at all locations. The news media items served to confirm the worth of our collegial relationships with community partners–and also proved to be the best introduction to new partners, as noted above.

To the extent possible, we provide training in the location and the situation in which it applies. In the reading program, we taught new tutors (community members) using a video made on location from real tutoring sessions, plus demonstrations with students and guided practice–usually in four 1-hr sessions with follow-up supervision (Power, Dowrick, Ginsburg-Block, & Manz, 1999). Where possible, new tutors were apprenticed until they reached 90% correct on the protocol.

Over time, experienced tutors became trainers. In the first 3 years, we trained nearly 50 community tutors in this way; four key master tutors had the main responsibility for training over half of them.

In the recess program, we identified a project coordinator (a community member, usually a current playground assistant) to help train other playground or lunchroom assistants in promoting children's social skills. This coordinator co-led fortnightly meetings with recess assistants, helped to collect integrity and outcome data, and assisted in solving problem situations.

Capacity Building with Community Partners– Responsibility and Empowerment

We build capacity of all participants to meet their own needs with their own resources. We were most successful in empowering community members in the following ways. The first neighborhood participants were identified by school staff. We gave them a place in the school, a place in the system, and specific responsibilities with the students. Later, they became the main source for new recruits. We provided highly specific skills training, in contrast to "could you help these children with their reading," which some of them had experienced previously as school volunteers (see *partner* vs. *delegate* models, Manz et al., 1999). For example, the tutors learned a routine for 25 minute step-by-step student interaction in which every contingency was covered. The playground partners were taught where to stand, what observations to make, and when and how to interact with students. They gradually assumed added roles and responsibilities: they collected data and entered it into computer files; they monitored and coached each other; and they chose activities and rewards for the children. We also found ways to support local values, language, and culture, and to address disabilities without the use of labels.

School staff were asked to provide models and to participate in problem solving. When they came to us for help with learning and behavior problems of individual students, we taught them a problem solving approach so they reached a solution *and* learned a new strategy for future use. Rather than solve health and mental health problems directly, we helped improve links with existing community resources. We taught the principles of self modeling and feedforward, shared information about phonics software and word games, and taught the associated uses of technology. Some community partners and parents also learned how to use the video and computer technology.

The parents were empowered by invitations to the school to see the individualized videos of their children or other new supports being provided. These reasons were positive–in contrast to being invited to school because the child is failing or a troublemaker. The opportunity was often taken to teach the parent how to support reading or positive social interactions at home. Some of these parents became volunteers in the school.

The capacity of students to succeed was enhanced by celebrating them as role models. They were featured in instructional videos, newspaper articles, and as partners in carefully selected groups. We held parties every term, so the students receiving special help could feel they were joining a club, rather than being singled out for failure. There were various rewards (stickers, food, game-time, praise) for trying hard or just for showing up, rather than for success in comparison with others.

Positive Visions–Creating Images of Future Success

Our philosophy-in-practice is built on positive images. Technology provided the most structured opportunities to create images of future success. In particular, we used *video futures* or feedforward (Dowrick, 1999) to boost children's reading. Short (2 min) videos were made to show students reading (relatively) fluently and recognizing a mix of common, but for them challenging, words on sight. These videos were made by practicing and staging selected passages for the camera, and by editing video footage from successful tutoring sessions. The students watched their images of "future capabilities" just prior to tutoring sessions. This approach was used for students making insufficient progress on tutoring alone, or after threats to self-efficacy, such as long absences from school or advancing to more difficult reading material (Kim-Rupnow, Galbavy, Anderson, & Dowrick, 1999).

We maximized the more general use of feedforward throughout all our programs (Power et al., 1999). For example, reading tutors and playground assisstants were taught minimal error correction. Words not attempted were prompted with a clue (beginning sound) and words misread were ignored so as never to interrupt a student's reading. Inconsiderate play was not punished, but new social skills, or a new game, were taught instead. Children were taught to see their progress in difficult tasks (e.g., reading fluently) by comparison with their own past performance, rather than by comparison with others (Bandura, 1997). The progress of community partners working in the schools was encouraged in the same way. For example, we held regular meetings with the playground staff, in which we showed graphical data, so staff could see their role in the improvements.

The empowerment roles described above contributed to positive visions. Community partners and students saw themselves and others of their number exercising leadership, showing progress, or being role models. We used reframing to support positive images. For example, we steered people away from the usual tendency to talk about the rate of "bad" behavior (e.g., running in the corridors) as negative data on what needed to be punished or prevented; we reframed these events as opportunities to teach social skills. When people negatively described what had been happening, they were asked to describe the positive alternatives they would like to see happening.

Data-Based Evaluation, Participatory Action Research

We take every opportunity to involve participants at all levels of research and action. The whole school community participated in the research, making it meaningful and responsive. The efforts to involve the school and its community in front end planning were difficult, as noted earlier. The schools wanted to see summaries of plans, to receive copies of everything (e.g., grant proposals), but to leave to us the efforts for securing and reporting external funding. Once the programs were tangibly underway, opportunities to be involved at all levels were widely embraced.

Continual efforts of communication were required. Data monitoring was extensive and rigorous. All students referred to the reading program were screened with individual assessments of reading level, IQ, teacher evaluations, and student self-reports. Once in the program, their progress was monitored with curriculum-based assessment of oral fluency twice a week. Tutors kept notes on every session, and all sessions were observed or tape recorded (Power et al., 1999). The playground was divided into zones, and independent observers recorded equipment availability and use, types of interactions among students, and any personnel actions (Leff et al., 1998). Data were collected from the school nurse and classroom teachers. Information summaries were discussed weekly with tutors and recess people, and quarterly with teachers, administrators, and community advisory groups (Leff et al., 1998).

Reactions and suggestions by participants led to continual revisions of the programs. For example, the reading tutoring protocols were changed ten times in the first 2 years. We then modified the system to add a phonemic awareness component–and added a variation to guide small group as well as individual tutoring. Reading a passage 'solo' twice rather than three times was advocated by a tutor, and the development of a memory game for sight words was suggested by a graduate student. A rotation of ethnically different games at recess was the suggestion of a community assistant. A student's request to show her futures video to her family led to the strategy of inviting parents into the school to observe videos and tutoring. It was a teacher's suggestion that one of our successful students with a cognitive disability become a tutor for a student in her class. And it was entirely at a family's initiative that one of our Vietnamese students teach her newly immigrated mother to read in English. We modified our interactions, training methods, and systems exposure in similarly extensive and diverse ways.

PRIMARY OUTCOMES

Protocol Development

Each of the programs described here made singular use of protocols to guide the instructional interactions of community partners with students. The ACE Reading program began with a 20 step protocol for tutoring that was at the core of training, tutoring, and evaluation. It helped anyone new to the program get a sense of what was involved. Trainee tutors used it as a 'cheat sheet' as they began to work with students, and all tutors were required to respond to it for immediate self-evaluation at the end of each session. This protocol was used for monitoring, feedback and feedforward, and for integrity and reliability checks. We revised it so often we relied on a version date and color coding to keep current. It provided a convenient basis for variations, such as group tutoring and use with different age students.

PLAYS began without a protocol because the situations were less structured. But the program made much slower progress than the reading program and we soon realized the significant contribution of the protocol. Despite a set of specific, conditional responses for playground supervision, the assistants' self-monitoring was very weak. Without self-monitoring and the expectation of other monitoring, intervention integrity deteriorated. We therefore developed a 10 item self-observation checklist, functionally comparable to the integrity checklist for the reading program.

Training and Other Program Assistant Outcomes

In 3 years, we trained over 50 reading tutors. By the third year, all new tutors were being trained primarily by an established lead tutor or Literacy Coordinator. All trainees were local community members, 95% were women, and 90% had children or grandchildren attending or recently attending the school. A large but imprecisely determined percentage were welfare recipients. Some trainees could evidently read at a primary grade level, while some had college degrees. Less than 10 were already employed in the school as educational assistants. All tutoring sessions were either observed by a colleague or were tape recorded. Tutoring matched the checklist protocols with 95% accuracy. Self-scoring of the checklists was verified, on a 20% sample of audiotapes, as also 95% accurate.

We made no attempt to screen candidates, therefore expecting some to drop out–which 20% did. One woman came to us as part of her welfare-to-work training. Some used the experience to build their resumes as a return to work or a stepping stone to enroll in college. One of our on-site coordinators reported:

> I supported two individuals in getting outside jobs. Others previously involved in the school expanded their service–leadership roles in the Parent Teacher Association and employed as Supportive Services Assistants. There were individuals from the neighborhood who had not been involved in the school prior to the project, many of whom became regulars, contributing greatly to the school as well as receiving the social rewards associated with helping children and making new friends. One great-grandmother, without any family enrolled in the school, became involved at the suggestion of a neighbor. Two women had daughters on the teaching staff. One had limited mobility, so we arranged for her to do her tutoring on the first floor and to have students come to her rather than for her to fetch them from the classroom.

Ten community partners were subsequently hired by the schools. We consider all these outcomes positive for the individuals concerned, and always made this view clearly understood–even though some of the outcomes may seem inefficient for the program.

We found that when a playground is divided into specific quadrants, providing structured games within a quadrant halved the amount of rough play and increased (3-fold) cooperative behavior (Leff et al., 1998). Structured games and active adult supervision both led to an increase in prosocial interactions among children of different ethnic backgrounds.

Student and Family Outcomes

Over 200 students received 40-80 tutoring sessions in the first 3 years of the reading program. The majority were in grade 1, with some in grades 2, 3 and 4. All were identified by teachers as in the bottom 15% of readers and otherwise at risk academically. Nearly 80% improved one or more reading grade levels and were considered able to function with their peers in class.

Parents and tutors reported positive changes in family lives, for example, turning off the TV after school, siblings reading to each other, or coaching reading using the same strategies as the tutors. Many students spent time at their neighborhood tutors' houses for additional social support.

School and Staff Outcomes

There have been widespread reports of staff-perceived improvements in reading generally, as well as for individual students, and in program satisfaction and related school harmony. There are also indications of improvements in parent perceptions of schools. As this article goes to press, we are collecting data related to these issues. There were a number of documented examples of individual students' improved attendance as a direct result of our programs.

System Outcomes

The three original schools adopted ACE Reading into their structure. Each school employed our lead tutor as a part-time coordinator, dedicated space to the program, and retained other community partners on an hourly basis. Funding continues through new grants and Title I or School Improvement budgets. One of our "clusters" of schools (K-12) adopted "literacy though technology and the fine and performing arts" for its new afterschool programs, influenced by ACE Reading.

The current PLAYS program includes social skills promotion and lunchroom organization, incentive systems, afterschool safety, and specific interventions for identified aggressors and victims.

Implementation and Adaptation

A large number of schools have undertaken the adaptation of ACE Reading. We have insisted on the key principles of positive visions and copious practice at the developmentally appropriate level, and the use of our procedures and protocols in some recognizable form. But we have also encouraged adaptations to the school's culture, educational philosophies, and strengths. Each program is renamed "The _____ (school or location name) ACE Reading Program." In two locations, neighborhood schools adopted the program by hiring tutors from our original schools as their coordinators. At press time, approximately 15 elementary schools, 7 middle schools, and 1 high school in three states were in the process of adapting and adopting the program. A "startup kit" is available, that includes manuals, videotapes, protocols, case studies, etc., (see www.cds.hawaii.edu/reading/).

The PLAYS recess program expanded from one to five urban schools in the district. It was cited as an example of Best Practice within Philadelphia in 1999.

CONCLUSIONS AND RECOMMENDATIONS

The greatest single lesson learned was the potency of capacity building with community individuals and organizations. They proved capable of delivering every aspect of their programs. They remained invested in their schools and communities. They ensured that services were culturally relevant and community responsive. And they could make a difference at an affordable cost. All factors described in our six element model made important contributions. In particular, these factors all supported the empowerment of our community partners. For example, establishing clear-cut, stable (but revisable) protocols and other written and electronic materials was essential to the successful training and the integrity of operation. Therein also lies the main hope for the maintenance of programs after the early players have gone. Flexibility is also important. If the right balance can be retained in allowing adaptations, encouraging ownership, and maintaining the integrity of the key features, there are sound prospects for increased implementation.

The programs are still undergoing a full economic analysis. It appears to cost (in 1999 US dollars) $10,000-$15,000 per year per school to bring most of the bottom 15% of first grade readers up to a participatory classroom level in moderate sized elementary schools in low income communities, although there are hidden costs in subsidizing the Coordinator, teacher time, etc. Costs may vary, depending on other factors such as home support (books, perceived importance of reading, etc.). These costs are far less than most alternative programs. Costs for the "Book Buddies" program appear to be comparable ($600 per student; Johnston, Invernizzi, & Juel, 1998) but programs using professional intervention specialists are six times as costly (Hiebert, 1994). The operational costs for PLAYS are similar to ACE Reading. The original programs altogether cost $700,000 to develop and evaluate; these costs are not factored into the current equations.

A word must be said about the role of technology, given that it provided much of the impetus for the research and development of these programs. The continuing lesson here has been the tantalizing promise of very significant effects tempered by the reality of a modest rate of adoption that is typical of technology in schools. Video seems to be very useful in jump-starting the response to tutoring. These outcomes were even more tantalizing given the obvious delight shown by most children in viewing their feedforward videos or in interacting with electronic games. Much of the selective attention of the press and of prospective adopters of the reading program is owed to the appeal of *feedforward.* Some students made exceptional progress in circumstances of tutoring plus video. Therefore we have subsequently pursued the simplification of feedforward technology with video and audiotape procedures, and begun the development of new computer software to automate the feedforward of reading (Dowrick & Kim-Rupnow, 1999).

There may have been contributing factors to the success of these programs, not applicable elsewhere, for example, the resources of the supporting institutions, and the personal contributions of individuals. And there were external barriers that may or may not exist in other settings. It seems likely that securing federal or large foundation grant support to establish new programs may add to their credibility with the community. Note our use of the term "empowerment" has been applied to individuals, not communities. We consider the schools to have become powerful in their own context but not in the free market. Unfortunately, with the approach offered by this model, communities remain economically poor and under-qualified in the larger context of society. Their success remains a type of subsistence, which can be changed only with a far greater shifting of resources and a much longer period of time.

A final caveat for prospective implementation: our model may be less applicable to better resourced communities, because there is less need and people are less hungry–did we make something work because of the (adverse) conditions, not despite them? It may take considerable adaptation to make these programs successful in wealthy suburbs or regions with traditions in reading at home. The resources and the underlying reasons for reading failure and school violence are so different in some communities that distinctively alternate strategies may be in order. We (the authors) are divided in this yet-to-be-tested speculation.

REFERENCES

Anderson, R.C. (1993). The future of reading research. In A.P. Sweet, & J.I. Anderson (Eds.). *Reading research into the year 2000.* Hillsdale, NJ: Lawrence Erlbaum.

Bandura, A. (1997). *Self-efficacy: The exercise of personal control.* New York: Freeman.

Black, M.M., & Krishnakumar, A. (1998). Children in low-income, urban settings: Interventions to promote mental health and well being. *American Psychologist, 53*, 635-646.

Chavis, D.M., Speer, P.W., Resnick, I., & Zippay, A. (1993). Building community capacity to address alcohol and drug abuse. In R. Davis & A. Lurigio (Eds.). *Drugs and the community: Involving community residents* (pp. 251-284). Springfield: Charles C Thomas.

Chung, H.H., & Elias, M. (1996). Patterns of adolescent involvement in problem behaviors: Relationship to self-efficacy, social competence, and life events. *American Journal of Community Psychology, 24*, 771-784.

Collins, H. (1997, October 27). Seeing is learning. *Philadelphia Inquirer,* pp. C1, C12.

Connell, J.P., Kubisch, A.C., Schorr, L.B., & Weiss, C. (1995). *New approaches to evaluating community initiatives.* Washington, DC: Aspen Institute.

Dowrick, P.W. (1998). A consideration of "community response programmes" for disabilities or other issues of common concern. *New Zealand Journal of Psychology, 27*(2), 30-35.

Dowrick, P.W. (1999). A review of self modeling and related interventions. *Applied and Preventive Psychology, 8,* 39-54.

Dowrick, P.W., & Kim-Rupnow, W.S. (1999). *Project I LIKE: Improving literacy by interacting with Kitten and Elephant.* Washington, DC: US Department of Education (awd #H327A990074).

Ginsburg-Block, M., & Fantuzzo, J. (1998). An evaluation of the relative effectiveness of NCTM standards-based interventions for low achieving urban elementary students. *Journal of Educational Psychology, 90,* 1-10.

Gresham, F. M., & Lopez, M. F. (1996). Social validation: A unifying concept for school-based consultation research and practice. *School Psychology Quarterly, 11,* 204-227.

Hawaii Department of Education. (1998). *Comprehensive assessment and accountability system.* Honolulu: Author.

Hiebert, E.H. (1994). Reading Recovery in the United States: What difference does it make to an age cohort? *Educational Researcher, 23,* 15-25.

Kim-Rupnow, W.S., Anderson, J., Galbavy, R., & Dowrick, P.W. (1999). *I Can Read! Self modeling to help young children with reading difficulties.* Manuscript submitted for publication.

Johnston, F.R., Invernizzi, M., & Juel, C. (1998). Book Buddies: Guidelines for volunteer tutors of emergent and early readers. New York: Guilford.

Leff, S.S., Costigan, T.E., Ginsburg-Block, M., Rudnicki, S., & Power, T.J. (1998, November). *The development of an observational coding system scheme to record aggressive and prosocial behavior and intercultural interactions on the playground.* Paper presented at annual conference of Association for Advancement of Behavior Therapy, Washington, DC.

Manz, P., Power, T.J., Ginsburg-Block, M., & Dowrick, P.W. (1999). *Community members as "community partners" in support of urban schools.* Manuscript submitted for publication.

Power, T.J., Dowrick, P.W., Ginsburg-Block, M., & Manz, P.H. (1999). *Building the capacity of urban schools to improve literacy skills: Community-assisted tutoring.* Manuscript submitted for publication.

Schorr, L.B. (1997). *Common purpose: Strengthening families and neighborhoods to rebuild America.* New York: Doubleday.

Tolan, P., Keys, C., Chertok, F., & Jason, L.A. (1990). *Researching community psychology: Issues of theory and methods.* Washington, DC: American Psychological Association.

University of Pennsylvania Library. (1998). http://www.library.upenn.edu/census/philschl/

US Census. (1990). Washington, DC: U.S. Government Printing Office.

White, G.W., Nary, D.E., & Froelich, A.K. (2001). Consumers as collaborators in research and action. *Journal of Prevention & Intervention in the Community, 21*(2), 15-34.

Wilson, W. (1996). *When work disappears: World of the new urban poor.* New York: Knopf.

Whyte, W.F. (Ed.). (1991). *Participatory action research.* Newbury Park, CA: Sage.

Zins, J.E. (Ed.). (1997). Community psychology contributions to consultation [special issue.] *Journal of Educational and Psychological Consultation, 8*(2).

Building Community
Coalitions with People
with Disabilities and Their Families:
An Empowerment Approach

Christopher B. Keys
Alan R. Factor

University of Illinois at Chicago

SUMMARY. How can community professionals help build coalitions that empower members of marginalized groups? The authors examine the building of rural, suburban, and urban coalitions on aging and developmental disabilities that sought to empower people with disabilities and their families. The coalitions addressed the four crucial issues of identifying local leaders, recruiting people with disabilities and family members, creating the chemistry of collaboration, and sustaining coalition activities. In order to empower members of marginalized groups, a critical mass of coalition leaders and members need to intend and then act to empower. Thirteen propositions are advanced concerning build-

Address correspondence to: Professor Christopher B. Keys, Department of Psychology MC 285, University of Illinois at Chicago, 1007 West Harrison Street, Chicago, IL 60607 <cbkeys@uic.edu>.

The authors appreciate the valuable contributions of project coordinator Eileen Gabriel and those of the community coalition members.

This research was funded by the Illinois Department on Aging through Grant No. 90AM0681 from the Administration on Aging, US Department of Health and Human Services, Washington DC 20101. The opinions expressed are those of the authors and not necessarily those of the funding agency.

[Haworth co-indexing entry note]: "Building Community Coalitions with People with Disabilities and Their Families: An Empowerment Approach." Keys, Christopher B., and Alan R. Factor. Co-published simultaneously in *Journal of Prevention & Intervention in the Community* (The Haworth Press, Inc.) Vol. 21, No. 2, 2001, pp. 91-112; and: *People with Disabilities: Empowerment and Community Action* (ed: Christopher B. Keys, and Peter W. Dowrick) The Haworth Press, Inc., 2001, pp. 91-112. Single or multiple copies of this article are available for a fee from The Haworth Document Delivery Service [1-800-342-9678, 9:00 a.m. - 5:00 p.m. (EST). E-mail address: getinfo@haworthpressinc.com].

91

KEYWORDS. Coalition building, empowerment, aging, developmental disabilities, disabilities

Many community psychologists and others concerned with the empowerment of people at the margins of society have recently recognized the value of community coalitions (Butterfoss, Goodman, & Wandersman, 1996). Coalitions can heighten community awareness of new and difficult social issues. They can bring disparate agencies and individuals together to propose and initiate broad-based community action. Coalitions have the potential to enable communities to work successfully on complex concerns that no agency or group could effectively consider alone (Gray, 1989).

Of fundamental importance to community professionals is coalition building to empower those who have less than reasonable access to society's resources. Moreover, coalitions are temporary systems that can benefit from the inclusion of members of marginalized groups who have direct knowledge of and experience with the convening social issue. However, while the value of such inclusion has been widely affirmed, less attention has been devoted to the central challenges in building community coalitions that empower. The primary purpose of this paper is to identify and illustrate four core issues of building empowering community coalitions. These issues are: (1) leadership, (2) member recruitment, (3) collaborative chemistry, and (4) sustaining activity. Each issue raises a distinctive challenge for empowering members of marginalized groups. We will address these issues and challenges from the point of view of the community professionals who are primarily responsible for initiating and facilitating coalitions during their beginning stages.

We will focus on three conditions necessary for the empowerment of marginalized group members through coalition building: (1) interest, (2) action and (3) impact (cf. Prilleltensky, 1999). For members of marginalized groups to become empowered coalition participants, all three conditions typically must be met. Also, coalition developers need to include members of marginalized groups. Within the last decade this intention has become more common among coalition builders. But given the long history of exclusion of marginalized persons from community development activities and the residual stigma in some quarters, it is important to make this intention explicit and central.

The second condition refers to taking action to promote the empowerment of persons at the margins. Action moves us beyond good intentions to taking steps to include and engage. The frequency, novelty, duration, and diversity of these actions contributes to their impact, the third condition necessary for empowerment. Intent and action, aligned and targeted, can have the impact of increasing the distinctive voices, meaningful choices, and influence of members of marginalized groups.

AGING AND DISABILITIES: THE EXEMPLAR OF COMMUNITY COALITION BUILDING

Our case exemplar is the development of three community coalitions to address issues of aging and developmental disabilities. The life expectancy of persons with developmental disabilities such as intellectual disabilities has lengthened considerably with greater awareness of the strengths of persons with disabilities, medical advances, and improved quality of life (Heller & Factor, 1993).

This increased longevity raises serious issues for people with developmental disabilities at middle age and beyond, including: obtaining supports for community living, dealing with aging parents, and planning for their lives after the death of their parents. Older parents may be concerned about how to support their adult child with a disability who in many cases lives with them. As their health declines, parents' concerns intensify as does the family's need for social services and later life planning. Agencies supporting persons with developmental disabilities have generally had little experience serving persons in middle age and beyond. As parents' needs increase, aging agencies often become the first to learn of the needs of older families with an adult child with disabilities. However, they have usually had scant experience serving families who have a member with developmental disabilities.

Recognizing these multiple concerns, the United States' Administration on Aging funded several model projects in the mid-1990s to develop community responses to the issues of aging and developmental disabilities. The model project described here had the goal of bridging aging and developmental disability networks to address community concerns. These concerns include educating service providers about local needs and resources, and increasing advocacy. Encouraging planning to prevent crises from occurring and facilitating access to services for older individuals with developmental disabilities and their families are also central. The authors were responsible for building three coalitions–one each in a rural, a suburban, and an urban community. These coalitions included older persons with developmental disabilities, older family caregivers of persons with developmental disabilities, aging social service agencies, disabilities agencies, and other relevant service and advocacy organizations.

LEADERSHIP

A major challenge in building empowering community coalitions is identifying and gaining the support of strong, effective, local leaders. These leaders have the ability to legitimize the coalition, its outside organizers, and the focal issue. In this case potential leaders have knowledge of and commitment to working on the issue of aging and developmental disabilities. They are also invested in empowering persons with developmental disabilities and their families. Without local leadership with these qualities, the future of the coalition is clearly compromised, especially when, as in the present case, the involvement of community professionals who are coalition builders is time limited.

How did coalition builders from outside the community identify and gain the support of local leaders in aging and developmental disabilities who were committed to empowering people with disabilities and their families? This is the empowerment challenge for leadership. First, we sought the direction and advice of the regional Area Agencies on Aging (AAA) to determine which local aging agencies they thought would be most likely to contribute to, and benefit from, participation in such a project. We hired a project coordinator who had been a staff member at a regional AAA and knew the aging delivery system and its key personnel. Based on our thirty years experience in the state working with agencies serving people with developmental disabilities, we also identified agencies and individuals in the disabilities field whom we believed could be empowering leaders in the communities recommended by the Area Agencies on Aging. Because of the dual focus on aging and developmental disabilities, we sought at least one lead agency from the aging network and one from the developmental disability network for each coalition.

We met with the prospective agency leaders identified in each of the three target communities to discuss coalition building in depth. During this meeting we shared information about issues of aging and developmental disabilities, and the concerns of older adults with developmental disabilities and their family caregivers. We asked about the degree of awareness and interest among community agencies in these issues. Then we exchanged views on the proposed local coalition–its empowering goals, and the roles of the lead agency, the coalition members, and the coalition organizers. We discussed the benefits of participating in the coalition and the support we would provide in initiating and facilitating coalition development.

We sought to determine the extent to which the agency could be likely to adopt an empowering stance toward people with developmental disabilities and their families. Regarding *intent*, we tried to ascertain whether the potential lead agencies agreed with an empowering approach to building community coalitions. Were they committed to building a coalition to address issues of aging and developmental disabilities that fully included persons with developmental disabilities and their family members in all coalition activities? Regarding *action*, we asked whether the potential lead agencies had a history of taking action to promote the empowerment of people with disabilities and their families. What kind of empowering actions had the agencies taken, e.g., support, advocacy, planning? Regarding *impact*, we asked about the results of prior efforts to promote empowerment. Had persons with disabilities and/or their families been fully included or in some other way increased their voice and influences as a result of agency efforts?

Thus, from background information, prior experience, and meetings, we determined the strengths and weaknesses of the potential lead agencies with regard to their likelihood of taking a strong empowering approach to coalition building. In general, the disability agencies had more experience with and were more attuned to the need for an empowering approach than the aging agencies. In the rural community of Plowshares, the prospective lead agency serving persons with developmental disabilities and their families was well respected in the community and thereby could help legitimize the proposed coalition. It had worked on disability and aging issues successfully. The agency's director was committed to taking a lead in building a community coalition on aging and developmental disabilities in which persons with developmental disabilities and family members would be welcome and involved. The agency had a history of action to support the development of advocates who were parents of youths with developmental disabilities. These actions had the impact of initiating a statewide training program for such advocates and having an advocacy program graduate as an agency staff member.

In contrast, the lead aging agency in Plowshares was less aware of empowerment issues. Nonetheless, the agency director indicated a commitment to aging issues of families with developmentally disabled members in both action and impact. She had a history of positive collaboration on these issues with the lead developmental disabilities agency. Overall then, Plowshares had the leadership potential to develop a strong, empowering coalition with positive agency ties, and commitment to the issue of interest.

In the suburban community of Riverbank, the developmental disabilities agencies were more committed to empowerment but less committed to participating in a community coalition than their rural counterpart. One had pioneered more inclusive community living for adults with developmental disabilities in the area. Another had developed a parent advocacy group that was perhaps the most effective in the state in its efforts to increase the awareness of public officials about disability services. Both agencies agreed to participate. But unlike Plowshares where the executive director and a key program manager provided leadership, in Riverbank direct service staff were the primary coalition members. Executive directors were available by phone and responsive to specific requests. While the developmental disabilities agencies were supportive of building an empowering community coalition, their commitments to their own growth and advocacy agenda took precedence and limited their coalition leadership efforts. One disability agency director indicated that agency directors would be unlikely to take part in a voluntary coalition when they could be pursuing other initiatives that would directly add "a million dollars" to their agency budget.

The two likely lead aging agencies in Riverbank were somewhat dubious about their responsibilities for serving persons with developmental disabilities and had little history of doing so. In fact, senior aging regional staff recommended Riverbank in part because they wanted these agencies to become more receptive to supporting older adults with developmental disabilities and their families. In Riverbank, there was at least distance, perhaps some distrust, and no pattern of past collaboration between the aging agencies and the developmental disabilities agencies. Finally, although willing to become engaged in coalition building, the aging agency leaders were unclear why a coalition was needed. They already participated in large interagency organization for general information sharing among more than 200 social service agencies in the area. That seemed to provide enough interagency interaction.

In Riverbank some elements for empowering leadership were initially evident, but others clearly were not. The developmental disabilities agencies' strong commitment to empowering persons with disabilities and their families was not matched by their commitment to aging issues or to coalition building. The aging agencies were ambivalent participants with little sign of intent, prior action or impact to demonstrate investment in empowering families of persons with developmental disabilities.

Consequently, there was space for other coalition leadership that local disability advocates and an advocacy agency filled quite effectively. These advocates had physical disabilities and a track record in advocating for disability rights. They enjoyed coalition building, had good relations with other disability advocates, and had had little prior contact with aging or developmental disability service providers.

In the urban Latino neighborhood of Calle Principal, leadership was tougher to find for the community coalition. The two primary agencies serving people with developmental disabilities had important strengths, but also had difficulty making leadership commitments. One large disability agency had pioneered innovative community support programs and been active in providing advocacy training for parents. It had made a strong effort to include persons with developmental disabilities on their board. It provided services to a large area of which the Calle Principal community was only a small part, at most 5%. The director assigned a part-time senior staff member to the coalition who was supportive but not knowledgeable about Calle Principal or Latino culture. The other agency focused on the local community offering a broad array of bilingual, bicultural social services for Latino children, youth, and adults with and without disabilities. It had a history of developing parent support and advocacy, followed by subsequent differences with advocates, and now little empowerment activity. The director assigned a bilingual Latino program manager to join the coalition who related well to parents but was often preoccupied with his own career issues.

The lead aging agency had good linkages with the Calle Principal neighborhood and had worked with other aging agencies there. It had a strong history of providing successful information dissemination programs and health screening for low income urban seniors. It had little history with developmental disabilities or empowerment, but because of a strong preexisting relationship with our project coordinator, an agency leader was open to an empowering approach and became committed to the coalition.

In short, in Calle Principal we had involvement from the disability agencies but not leadership, and leadership from the aging agency, but not knowledge of the issues or a background of empowerment. Initially, project staff provided more leadership and eventually we identified a group of older Latino parents with adult children with developmental disabilities living at home. These older parents became very involved with the urban coalition and provided substantial energy and direction for it.

From the foregoing, four propositions emerge for identifying potential coalition leaders who are committed to empowerment:

Proposition 1:   Good potential leaders intend to empower members of marginalized groups. They take action to promote such empowerment. They have a history of previous empowerment efforts that have had a positive impact in the lives of members of marginalized groups.

Proposition 2:   Good potential coalition leaders have a commitment to the convening issues of the coalition. They have direct knowledge of, and have been involved in activities to address these issues.

Proposition 3:   Good potential coalition leaders are connected to the community–its language, culture, people, and agencies. They have positive history of ongoing relationships with individuals and agencies who would join the coalition.

Proposition 4:   Good potential coalition leaders believe that building an empowering community coalition is an excellent way to address the convening issues. Top agency and group leaders commit to investing time in leading local coalition-building efforts.

These propositions point the way toward identifying effective coalition leaders. Yet as the examples make clear, it is quite unlikely that all leaders will satisfy or even approximate these ideals. We used these four guidelines to identify the best available lead agencies in developmental disabilities and aging. Where the agencies fell short, we sought help from other community members, and invested more staff time.

RECRUITMENT

Having identified coalition leaders, community professionals work with local leaders to address the next challenge: recruiting coalition members. Recruitment of representatives from diverse constituencies who, like the leaders, are generally supportive of an empowerment approach, interested in the convening issues, and invested in coalition work is essential to coalition success. Only with people from different constituencies contributing their distinctive perspectives in a climate of mutual respect can a coalition realize its goals of developing and acting effectively on complex, convening issues. Our recruitment approach involved asking the lead agencies to identify such potential coalition participants from their local networks of organizations and individuals. Project staff conducted additional grassroots community outreach where necessary to find possible participants. In meeting with potential participants, lead agencies, and project staff, we presented a clear vision of the coalition as planned, the role of coalition members, and the benefits of participating. We discussed potential members' interest in taking an empowering approach to addressing aging and developmental disabilities. Because some declined to participate and some participants left their coalitions, we found recruitment to be an ongoing process requiring open communication between coalition organizers and lead agencies and groups. In short, the empowerment challenge in recruiting is: How can coalition organizers and leaders find and recruit members of marginalized groups who are likely to become contributing members of the coalition?

In the rural community of Plowshares, the local lead agencies took primary responsibility for recruiting. Through their strong networks, they successfully recruited three local agencies serving primarily persons with developmental disabilities and their families and three local agencies serving older persons. Given the rural context, the lead agencies recruited widely, they involved four local social service agencies that were generally responsible for transportation, public health, public assistance, and housing for those in need. In addition, two regional agencies, one concerned with social service planning, and one with aging services agreed to participate.

Central to the empowering approach is recruiting individuals with developmental disabilities and their older family members. The lead developmental disabilities agency in Plowshares readily committed to recruiting families and persons with developmental disabilities and identified potential recruits. Agency leaders took full responsibility for the recruitment process and insured that an agency staff member discussed the coalition in understandable terms with each prospective recruit. The staff member asked recruits about what supports they would find helpful to their full participation in coalition activities, (e.g., transportation, respite services, coaching), and agreed to help with needed arrangements. These recruitment actions had a clear positive impact. From the first meetings three self-advocates with developmental disabilities and four family members were involved in the Plowshares coalition.

In suburban Riverbank, local leadership took longer to crystallize, resulting in somewhat slower recruitment efforts. Lead agencies recruited about a third of the coalition members and recommended other possible participants. Project staff followed up on these recommendations and pursued their own contacts to identify the rest. The coalition included seven local agencies that served people with developmental and other kinds of disabilities and one regional and four local aging services agencies. Again, the lead developmental disabilities agencies were more involved than aging agencies in nominating persons with developmental disabilities and their families. Project staff then contacted these individuals to discuss the coalition, their interests, and needed supports.

One developmental disabilities lead agency identified as prospective coalition members several persons with developmental disabilities who lived in community living arrangements that the agency managed. Initially, one of the home managers and a person with a communication disability had concerns that the role of persons with disabilities in the coalition would be more for appearance than for meaningful participation. Two project staff met with the person with a disability and staff member to get better acquainted with one another and to discuss the plans for the coalition in depth. The person with the developmental disability demonstrated how she could use her communication board to contribute meaningfully to the meetings. The person with the disability decided to join the coalition and the home manager consistently provided necessary transportation and meeting supports. After 6 months (in contrast to 2 months in Plowshares), 6 self-advocates with disabilities and 4 family members were participating in the Riverbank coalition.

In urban Calle Principal, the committed lead agency served seniors, but not persons with developmental disabilities. The agency leader suggested aging agencies who might join the coalition. Project staff pursued a number of his leads as well as contacting disability and aging agencies known to them. These efforts garnered nine aging agencies (seven local and two regional), and five disability agencies (two local and three regional) as coalition members.

A particular challenge was recruiting persons with developmental disabilities and their family members. Participating developmental disabilities agencies had few suggestions. The empowerment of Latinos with developmental disabilities was not a priority where many were already confronting issues of discrimination, restrictive immigration policies, cultural differences, and poverty. To find older families with a member with developmental disabilities, we visited churches, senior citizen centers, and public housing for seniors. Eventually our persistence was rewarded when a local politician told us of a group of parents with adult children with developmental disabilities who met weekly at his community office.

After a presentation by, and discussion with project staff, several families from this parent group agreed to join the coalition. Following cultural norms, parents rather than persons with developmental disabilities typically participated. Strong involvement was empowering for parents, but there was little direct opportunity to address the empowerment of persons with disabilities.

Thus, recruitment is the first litmus test of the commitment of the lead agencies to building an empowering coalition. Vitally important are the leaders' intent, action, and impact in recruiting persons with disabilities and their families. Lead agencies and project staff were ultimately successful in recruiting a sizable cohort of persons with disabilities and family members for each coalition. Yet the role of the lead agencies in this important step toward empowerment varied greatly. In the rural community of Plowshares, developmental leaders conducted the entire recruitment process with minor technical support from project staff. In suburban Riverbank, the lead disability agencies involved worked as helpful partners recruiting one third of the persons with disabilities and suggesting others. In urban Calle Central, the project staff were responsible with minor help from developmental disabilities agencies and some assistance and encouragement from a leader of an aging agency.

We advance the following propositions concerning the recruitment of persons with developmental disabilities and their families into coalitions:

Proposition 5:   Leaders with ties to those sought are valuable for successful recruitment. Agencies with stronger leadership qualities as defined in prior propositions will put forth greater recruiting effort and have more success than other agencies.

Proposition 6:   Recruiting at least three persons with disabilities and three family members is necessary for these members of previously marginalized groups to be comfortable, contributing members of a coalition.

THE CHEMISTRY OF COLLABORATION

Once leaders have been selected and members have been recruited, then the third challenge of coalition building emerges–developing a chemistry of collaboration among coalition members. Collaborative processes are essential to bringing multiple constituencies together–first to develop shared plans and then to enact them successfully. One way to develop momentum for empowering collaboration is to respect and support the varying perspectives of different constituencies (cf. Bartunek, Foster-Fishman, & Keys, 1996). In the present project once persons with disabilities and family members joined the coalitions, we initiated a participatory planning process that enabled each person to introduce themselves, discuss their interests concerning aging and developmental disabilities, and indicate what they considered to be the high priority local needs concerning aging and developmental disabilities.

For assessing local needs, we used a group-building approach that began with individuals reflecting on community needs. Then participants shared their priorities in small groups of 3 or 4 persons and chose one that was the most important, one most urgent, and one most likely to galvanize community support. As the small groups offered their priority issues to the large group, the community facilitator worked with members to organize the various issues by content area, e.g., education, transportation, advocacy, housing, and employment. Then coalition members voted for their top three choices from among the content areas represented. Members discussed the two to five priorities they had endorsed the most and decided which ones they wanted to form action groups to address. Overall this process took three or four monthly meetings of two to three hours duration. Coalition organizers allowed ample time for each member to have input, and to reflect and comment on the needs identified and endorsed. In each community this process resulted in clarifying participants' commitment to the coalition, building relationships among coalition members, establishing priorities, and organizing groups to take action on them.

Next, the action groups and the entire coalition specified major initiatives they wanted to undertake. Initially, action groups sought to identify a particular initiative that addressed their priority area and galvanized member commitment. Regularly scheduled meetings were held to build momentum for working on the initiatives. Additional opportunities to interact by phone, e-mail, and face-to-face between meetings strengthened collaborative norms and members' ties to the coalition. We also found it important to be flexible and responsive to member feedback about coalition processes. How meetings are conducted, when they are scheduled, and how coalition organizers, leaders and members interact were all considered and improved by responding to member feedback. The successful completion of an initiative provided participating coalition members a sense of accomplishment and motivation for further coalition activities. In sum, planning and conducting meaningful, successful initiatives in an open, participatory way can establish the chemistry of collaboration that builds the strength of the community coalition.

Establishing the chemistry of collaboration raised two empowerment questions with action implications. First, how could leaders act to fully include people with developmental disabilities and their families in the needs assessment process? Second, how could leaders act to help people with disabilities and family members find meaningful roles that contribute to coalition initiatives?

In rural Plowshares, the needs assessment process included active participation of persons with developmental disabilities and their families. The local lead developmental disabilities agency recruited effectively, provided transportation and respite care, and helped to schedule the meetings so that self advocates and family members could attend. The agency staff met with persons with developmental disabilities prior to the coalition sessions. Staff explained the needs assessment process and gave persons with disabilities time in advance to think about the issues, discuss their relevant experience, and prepare what they wanted to contribute to the discussion of coalition priorities. The lead developmental disabilities agency also arranged for staff to support participants during coalition meetings. Staff sat next to and encouraged individuals with disabilities to contribute to group discussions. Staff also helped all participants recognize when meeting discourse was overly complex and rapid, so that they could speak in a way all members understood. As a result of the developmental disabilities agency's effective provision of support and the coalition organizers participatory planning approach, persons with disabilities and their families were actively involved in the needs assessment of the Plowshares coalition.

In Plowshares developing coalition initiatives involved efforts to find meaningful roles for participants with developmental disabilities and their families. The rural coalition established transportation and education as its priorities and formed two action groups, one to develop an initiative for each priority. The transportation action group sought to ascertain the nature and extent of transportation needs by surveying people with developmental disabilities and their families in the county. The participation of action group members with developmental disabilities and family members was instrumental. They shaped the content of the questionnaire, the strategy of data gathering in governmental and not-for-profit agency offices, the interpretation of the results, and the recommendations for action (e.g., agency support for informal car pools). This involvement of persons with disabilities and their families strengthened the quality of the survey from initial inception to final results.

The action group for education focused on informing aging, and, to a lesser extent, developmental disabilities service providers about developmental disabilities and aging issues, services, and other resources in the region. The group obtained funding from the Area Agency on Aging to host a major training event on these issues which attracted 70 staff from social service agencies in a sixteen-county region around Plowshares. One very positive part of this training session was an address by a coalition member with developmental disabilities on issues facing middle-aged adults with developmental disabilities and their older parents. Participants considered her talk an informative highlight. Developmental disabilities agency staff supported her in preparing and practicing this talk. Having a meaningful role mobilized this speaker's commitment to the coalition. It also increased other coalition members' appreciation of the strengths she could offer. Following this success, she became a central member of the coalition and made important contributions to other activities.

In Riverbank local advocates with physical disabilities helped provide leadership and increased the voice and influence of people with disabilities. Two of the local advocates were distinctly talented, experienced individuals who readily assumed active roles on the coalition and provided models for involvement of persons with disabilities. Having two developmental disability agencies with a commitment to empowering persons with disabilities and their families helped establish a positive chemistry of collaboration. Agency and project staff acted on this intention to empower by providing support for inclusion for members with developmental disabilities including transportation, meeting preparation, and facilitation of meeting involvement. They encouraged all persons with disabilities and family members to become as fully involved as possible. The impact of these actions was that the two talented, experienced members with disabilities became central to this suburban coalition. Their active participation helped make full involvement of people with disabilities a coalition norm. For example, coalition members also became attuned to involving an individual who used a communication board to interact. In short, not all coalition members were initially aware of or committed to the empowerment of people with disabilities and their families. Yet enough leaders were so committed that they engaged both individuals with disabilities and family members in needs assessment.

These actions to empower people with disabilities during project planning had a positive impact on the subsequent activities of the

Riverbank coalition. During needs assessment, the group identified education as top priority and decided to pursue two projects. The leader of a disability organization recommended advocacy training for people with disabilities. This specific project attracted most of the attention of members with disabilities. Coalition members with disabilities were very active in planning, conducting, and receiving advocacy training. They helped choose the curriculum topics (e.g., learning to write advocacy letters), recruit speakers (e.g., government officials), organize logistics (e.g., scheduling sessions so participants can take buses to and from training), and recruit personal care attendants for participants. Two members with disabilities and one parent gave presentations on advocacy tactics, local disability advocacy organizations, and the history of disability advocacy; they also facilitated group discussions. Four other coalition members with disabilities participated in and reported benefitting from the advocacy training. In brief, the Riverbank coalition enjoyed success in empowering persons with disabilities. The intentions and actions to empower by coalition leaders and staff and the positive qualities of the members with disabilities were important in making the chemistry of collaboration effective.

In urban Calle Principal, the commitment to empowering family members with disabilities was held primarily by project staff. Eight Spanish-speaking parents with adult children with developmental disabilities became core members of the coalition. We scheduled coalition meetings for mid-morning, after their adult children had gone to vocational programs and before they returned home in the afternoon. Bilingual project and agency staff helped conduct meetings in both English and Spanish. These actions and parents' reliable attendance had the initial impact of giving them a major voice in identifying local needs. They focused on the need for more information about available social and health services and government programs (e.g., social security).

To address this need, the coalition members decided to hold a local information fair primarily for families of adults with developmental disabilities. Coalition members invited the area social service and health agencies and government programs to participate. An aging agency leader with experience in conducting information fairs encouraged parents to become involved in the project. Parents distributed flyers about the fair to neighborhood churches, senior housing centers, and businesses. They encouraged past and present members of their support group to attend. Their promotion efforts contributed significantly to recruiting approximately 100 family members, people with disabilities and interested others to attend the fair.

In Calle Principal the project staff's commitment to empower parents led to action that spanned barriers of cultural and class differences. Although few local agency leaders were providing support for parent empowerment, the efforts of project staff and the aging agency leader were sufficient to have a noticeable positive impact.

Overall, the empowerment challenge in establishing the chemistry of collaboration is one of inclusion and involvement. The primary focus here is aligning intent and action to effectively include persons with disabilities and their families in coalition activities. Based on the experiences of these three coalitions, we offer the following propositions concerning empowerment through inclusion:

Proposition 7:   Coalition leaders and staff must have a commitment to the inclusion of members of marginalized groups for it to happen. This commitment need not be made by all leaders and staff but by enough to make effective action possible.

Proposition 8:   For persons with disabilities and their families to become included, coalition members and staff must provide appropriate supports. These supports must be individually tailored to the needs of the individuals to be included.

Proposition 9:   Finding meaningful roles in the coalition for people with disabilities and their families involves both their willingness to participate and encouragement of their participation by some other coalition members (cf. Foster-Fishman & Keys, 1997).

Proposition 10:   Once included with active voices and meaningful roles, persons with disabilities and their families use their talents to improve the work of the coalition.

SUSTAINING COALITION INVOLVEMENT

The success of coalition projects creates a momentum to continue the work of the coalition. Nonetheless, voluntary coalitions can be fragile. The loss of coalition organizers and outside funding can be sufficient to end the coalition and its capacity for empowerment. Over time a coalition inevitably faces transitional issues including leadership succession, planning new activities, and obtaining resources. The empowerment challenge here is: How can persons with disabilities and their family members be encouraged to continue their investment in the coalition over time?

In rural Plowshares, agency leaders, project staff, and coalition members discussed a major transition. After two years, external funding would cease and project staff would be available only for limited consultation, not for ongoing operational support and coordination. The coalition members met and decided to continue the coalition. The lead disability agency agreed to provide staff to coordinate the coalition. To enact this good intention, coalition members arranged several activities. First, they organized a training session on an issue of great importance to aging parents and adult children with developmental disabilities, viz., legal guardianship. They invited a leading national attorney on guardianship and disabilities to speak in Plowshares. Second, with the assistance of project staff, they prepared a grant proposal to promote the full inclusion of older people with disabilities into community life. Third, the coalition held an orientation session for area social service staff and families on new housing options that encouraged people with disabilities to live as independently as possible in the community.

In all these important activities, coalition members with disabilities and family members were involved. They shaped the setting of coalition priorities. They helped promote the guardianship training program. They provided ideas for the grant proposal on community inclusion. One coalition member with a developmental disability provided a tour of her apartment for participants in the housing seminar to illustrate the new community living options. In short, the Plowshares coalition sustained itself through planning collaboratively, having lead agencies accept more leadership responsibility, and initiating valued new activities. Throughout this transition the coalition members reaffirmed their intention to empower by acting to include persons with developmental disabilities and their families and by making their concerns a coalition priority.

In suburban, blue collar Riverbank, there was less overall investment in the coalition by agency leaders and an even stronger commitment to empowerment by agency staff than in Plowshares. Fortunately, in the closing months of the federal funding, a new aging agency leader joined the coalition who was more committed to sustaining the coalition in some form. She led the coalition in discussions to consider becoming part of a large local interagency planning council.

Core coalition members with disabilities were central to these discussions and raised a number of concerns about joining the council. These concerns were productively discussed with a number of council members. Council members were receptive to having the coalition merge with a relevant council committee. Their receptivity was based in part on a presentation about the coalition made by a member who was the parent of an adult child with a developmental disability. Constructive discussions enabled both groups to talk through their concerns, and develop the foundation of trust necessary for including the coalition in the structure of the interagency council. At last report this merger was proceeding positively.

The Riverbank coalition's strong prior record of empowerment of people with disabilities and their family members shaped assumptions about the roles of these empowered members. It was assumed that people with disabilities and family members would participate fully and they did. It was as if the three-step cycle of intention, action, and impact had previously been so empowering that the particulars of each of these steps now were less important. The coalition's successful work with empowerment transformed these three, initially separate steps, into a single norm for including persons with disabilities and families as full, valued coalition participants. Their empowered involvement had become a natural, accepted part of coalition functioning.

In urban Calle Principal sustaining the coalition was problematic because of the limited agency leadership. Project staff worked with parents and agency staff to plan future directions. Parents identified the problem of aging neighbors with adult children with disabilities who were isolated and unaware of available community social agencies and other supports. A local disability agency tentatively agreed to serve as a base of operations for a new initiative of outreach to older Latino families with adult children with disabilities. Project staff identified an interested funder who agreed to consider paying parents to work part-time as community outreach staff. Subsequently, parent leaders grew apprehensive about the commitment required of them, their safety in conducting community outreach and the uncertainty of support from an agency that had not been an active coalition participant. The parents ultimately decided not to pursue development of the outreach project, but to suspend coalition activities.

In Calle Principal, parents were highly empowered. Over time, they became the most active members. Ultimately, they decided the future of the coalition. They had become empowered in the coalition in the absence of major involvement by local agencies. Consequently, when the project funding ceased, there were insufficient trusted agency and interagency resources available to help sustain a coalition. The collaboration necessary for successful coalition activity was adequate when supported by project staff, but not when responsibility for ongoing operations was to be transferred to local coalition members (cf. Bond & Keys, 1993).

Overall, the empowerment processes set in motion earlier in the life of a coalition affect how a coalition later sustains itself. In Plowshares people with disabilities and their families had been empowered through meaningful participation. They participated in planning and conducting activities to sustain their coalition. In Riverbank people with disabilities had become influential coalition members. They had a major impact on negotiations to restructure the coalition. In Calle Principal parents of adults with developmental disabilities became more empowered as the investment of agency personnel wavered over time. The parents ultimately decided the fate of the coalition.

The following propositions concerning sustaining community coalitions are worthy of reflection and empirical examination:

Proposition 11: Successful experience with empowering people with disabilities and family members can lead to the establishment of coalition norms for their full involvement in the life of the coalition.

Proposition 12: Sustaining an empowering community coalition requires committed leaders, empowered members from constituencies at the margins of society, and a chemistry of collaboration between them.

Proposition 13: In communities with fewer material resources it may be more difficult to sustain coalition activities following the withdrawal of external funding.

CONCLUSION

This paper examines the processes of empowerment of people with disabilities and their family members in three community coalitions concerned with issues of aging and developmental disabilities. To the authors' knowledge it is the first paper to examine how such marginalized individuals may become empowered in community coalitions. This perspective identifies four major issues in building empowering community coalitions. First, the results of these coalition-building efforts indicate the crucial importance of coalition leadership that is committed to empowering marginalized members in both intent and impactful action. The present examples indicate the value of identifying these local coalition leaders, and the necessity for community psychologists and other professionals to provide leadership for empowerment when such local leaders are unavailable.

Second, leaders' proactive recruitment of multiple marginalized members is necessary if these members are to make a difference in the coalition. We recommend that at least 35% of the active members of the coalition be members of marginalized groups. Third, coalition leaders' commitment to the inclusion of marginalized members in coalition meetings and activities is crucial to these members' full involvement. Empowering leaders provide individualized supports, expect significant participation and help develop meaningful roles for members of marginalized groups who desire to contribute. These empowered members can then distinctively contribute to the success of coalition activities. Fourth, the continuing involvement of effective local leaders and empowered members of marginalized groups are both important to sustaining coalition activities following the end of external funding and the reduction of involvement by community professionals. In communities with fewer resources, the withdrawal of external grant support for coalition building may be more difficult to overcome.

In addressing each of these four crucial issues, we found that community professionals needed to find and work with coalition members who articulated the intent to empower members of marginalized groups. These members needed to be skilled enough to act effectively on their intent to have an empowering impact. For each challenge we saw that taking effective action based on positive intent was the path to achieve empowering impact. Riger (1993) has noted that too often empowerment rhetoric raises expectations but does not lead to action or become a reality for those living in the shadows of society. Tightly coupling intent, action, and impact is an antidote for the loose use of the empowerment construct.

REFERENCES

Bartunek, J., Foster-Fishman, P., & Keys, C. (1996). Using collaborative advocacy to foster intergroup cooperation: A joint insider-outsider investigation. *Human Relations, 49*, 701-733.

Bond, M., & Keys, C. (1993). Empowerment, diversity and collaboration: Promoting synergy on community boards. *American Journal of Community Psychology, 21*, 37-57.

Butterfoss, F., Goodman, R., & Wandersman, A. (1996). Community coalitions for prevention and health promotion: Factors predicting satisfaction, participation and planning. *Health Education Quarterly, 23*, 65-79.

Foster-Fishman, P., & Keys C. (1997). The person environment dynamics of employee empowerment: An organizational culture analysis. *American Journal of Community Psychology, 25*, 345-370.

Gray, B. (1989). *Collaborating: Finding common ground for multiple party problems.* San Francisco: Jossey-Bass.

Heller, T., & Factor, A. (1993). Support systems, well being and placement decision-making among older adults and their children with developmental disabilities. In E. Sutten, A. Factor, B. Hawkins, T. Heller & G. Seltzer (Eds.), *Older adults with developmental disabilities: Optimizing choice and change.* Baltimore: Brookes.

Prilleltensky, I. (1999). *Participatory processes in community action: Partnerships to promote child wellness.* Presentation at the Interamerican Congress of Psychology, Caracan, Venezuela.

Riger, S. (1993). What's wrong with empowerment? *American Journal of Community Psychology, 21*(3), 279-292.

Index

ACE Reading program. *See also* Community Response Model
  capacity-building with community partners, 80-81
  data-based evaluation and participatory action research, 82-83
  establishing a place in the system, 78-79
  expansion to other schools, 86
  identification of needs and strengths, 77-78
  outcomes, 83-86
  positive visions, 81-82
  working relationship–a resource to the community, 79-80
Action Letter Portfolio, 23-27. *See also* Participatory Action Research
  need for advocacy letter writing skills, 22,24
  description of, 22-23
  dissemination of, 25-26
  effectiveness of, 25-26
  evaluation of, 26-27
Action groups. *See* community empowerment
Administration on Aging, 93
Adventuresome research methods and evaluation, 12
Advocacy. *See also* self-advocacy
  and independent living goals, 4,25-26
  and Latinos with disabilities, 67
  need for, 39-40
  and people with chronic fatigue syndrome, 39-40
  and people with developmental disabilities, 96
  risks of, 64
Advocacy action-planning guide, 64. *See also* Community empowerment
Advocacy and Organizational Development Group, 56
Aging,
  Administration on Aging, 93
  Area Agencies on Aging (AAAs), 94
  with a developmental disability, 93-94,95
  and life-expectancy, 93
Americans with Disabilities Act (ADA)
  advocacy efforts by Latinos with disabilities, 54-68
  enforcement of/compliance with, 22,26,55,57
  passage of, 3,18
  National Council on Disability hearings, 55-56
  and minorities with disabilities, 55
American Disabled for Attendant Programs Today (ADAPT), 17-18

Bell, Alexander Graham, 16
Best practices, 72,74,86

Capacity-building. *See* community empowerment approach to capacity-building
Centers for independent living, 26,56
Centers for Disease Control, 38
Civil Rights Act of 1964, 55
Change agents, *see* community empowerment

Chicago Chronic Fatigue Syndrome
    Association, 38-44,48
Children with disabilities. *See also*
    Education for all Children's
    Act and Individuals with
    Disabilities Education Act
  advocacy efforts by parents of, 56
  education of, 3,4,55
Chronic fatigue syndrome. *See also*
    Ecological approach to
    community collaboration
  and advocacy efforts, 39-40
  attitudes toward, 39,40
    by physicians, 39,44
  and daily assistance, 45-47
    Buddy/Mentor intervention,
      46-47
  Chicago Chronic Fatigue Syndrome
    Association, 38-44,48
  children with, 47-48
  and community psychology,
    37,45,49
  and the value of an ecological
    approach, 42,44,47
  and employment, 40-42
    development of a job bank, 41-42
  epidemiology of, 38
  etiology of, 37,49
  and housing/independent living,
    42-45
    shared housing programs, 43-44
  and illness management, 46
    energy conservation model, 46
    global measure of expended
      energy, 45-46
  Medical Professionals/persons with
    CFS, 38
  needs assessment, 39-40
  nurses with, 38
  prevalence of, 37,38
  and public policy, 37-38,45
  recovery from, 39
  resource directory for, 47
  within a socio-political context, 39
  and self-help groups, 40,42-46,48
    and university collaborators,
      48-49
  and stigma, 37,39
  symptoms of, 37
  treatment of, 39,49-50
    role of community psychologists
      in, 49-50
Coalition building, 92-112
  in Calle Principal, 97-98,101-102,
    106-107,109-110
  challenges to, 94,96
  chemistry of collaboration, 102-107
    propositions for a successful
      chemistry of collaboration,
      107
  conditions necessary for, 92
  fragility of coalitions, 107
  group-building approach, 103
  leadership, 94-99
    propositions for successfully
      identifying coalition leaders,
      98-99
  and marginalized groups, 92-93,
    111-112
  membership recruitment, 99-102
    propositions for successful
      recruitment of coalition
      participants, 102
  needs assessment, 104,106
  in Plowshares, 95-96,99-100,
    104-105,108
  in Riverbank, 96-97,100-101,
    105-106,108-109
  sustaining activity, 107-110
    propositions for successfully
      sustaining community
      coalitions, 110
  value of, 92
Coalition Building Model, 7,9-10
Collaboration. *See also* Ecological
    approach to collaboration
    and Participatory Action
    research
  between researcher and participant,
    16,21,36,48
Community coalitions, *see* Coalition
    building

Community Collaboration Model, 7,10-11
Community empowerment, 54,66-67
  capacity-building approach to, 57
  change agents, 57,58,61,63,66-67
  limitations of, 67-68
  phases of a capacity building
    approach to community
    empowerment, 57-58
    community entry, 59-60
      barriers to, 59
    community organizing, 61-62
      and action groups, 61
      barriers to, 62
    identifying strengths and
      concerns, 60-61
      barriers to, 60
      Concerns Report Method, 60
      and focus groups, 60-61
    monitoring/feedback, 63-64
      advocacy action-planning
        guide, 64
    planning and taking action,
      62-63
      ADA action groups, 62-63
      action logs, 62
      barriers to, 62-63
    sustaining community
      organizing methods, 64,66
  to promote independent living
    goals among people with
    disabilities, 55
  utility of, 67
Community Psychology, 2,12,39,45
  and disability studies, 2,5,11-12
  and epidemiological research,
    37,49
  and "people in trouble," 5,49,92
  principles of, 5,11,54,73
  tensions,
    between research rigor and
      procedural flexibility, 73
    between research rigor and
      relevance, 20,21
    between social action and
      scientific skepticism, 4,12

  and under resourced communities,
    72
Community responsiveness,
  general model of, 5-6
  models of, 5-11
Community Response Model,
  7-8,72-88
  barriers to, 87
  capacity-building, importance of,
    86
  and community stakeholders, 73-74
  cost of, 86,87
  and empowerment, 75,86,88
  feedforward, 75,80,81,87
  positive visions, 75-76
  and school interventions, *see* ACE
    Reading program and
    PLAYS Recess program
  six element approach to,
    capacity-building with
      community partners, 75
    data-based evaluation and
      participatory action research,
      76
    establishing a place in the
      system, 74
    identification of needs and
      strengths, 73-74
    working relationship–a resource
      to the community, 74-75
  and sustainability, 73,86
  in under resourced communities,
    72,77
    versus better resourced
      communities, 88
  utility for diverse populations, 75
Constituent validity, 11, *See also*
  Kelly, James
Consumers, 16-32,67,72-86
  See also people with disabilities
  as collaborators, *see also* Consumer
    Response Model,
    Coalition-building *and*
    Participatory Action
    Research

Demonstrations, 18
Department of Disability and Human
    Development, 56
Developmental disabilities,
    and advocacy, 94,95,97
    aging with a developmental
        disabilities, 93-94,95
    empowerment of people with,
        92-112. *See also*
        Coalition-building
    and longevity, 93
Disabled people. *See* People with
    disabilities
Disability rights movement, 2,3-4,12
Disability studies, 2,3-4,11
    and community psychology,
        2,5,11-12
    and the disability rights movement, 3
    tensions,
        between social action and
            scientific skepticism, 4,12
Discrimination. *See* Chronic fatigue
    syndrome, minorities with
    disabilities, *and* people with
    disabilities

Ecological approach to community
    collaboration
    Citizen advisory groups, 36
    and collaborative relationships,
        36,40
    and people with chronic fatigue
        syndrome, *see* Chronic
        Fatigue Syndrome
    and people with disabilities, 50
    principles of, 36-37
    and sustainability, 36
    value of, 42,50
Ecological model, 36,40,50. *See also*
    Kelly, James
Education of all Children Act, 3
Emancipatory research, 4
Empowering community coalitions,
    see Coalition building
Empowerment, 5,9-10,75,111-112

See also Coalition-building
See also Community empowerment
See also Rappaport, Julian
See also Riger, Stephanie
    definition of, 54
    limitations of, 111-112
    principles of, 63
    and Participatory Action Research,
        16
    role of the professional, 67,92

Feedforward, 75,80,81,87
    See also Community Response
        Model, and technology, uses
        of

Grassroots outreach, 99

Individuals with Disabilities Education
        Act (IDEA), 3,56
    and minority children with
        disabilities, 56
Interventions,
    real-life application, 21
    school-based, *see* ACE Reading
        program and PLAYS Recess
        Program
    sustainability of, 20,36,73

Kelly, James, 11,36

Latino(a)s with disabilities
    advocacy efforts, 55
    capacity building approach to
        community empowerment
        with Latino(a)s with
        disabilities, 54-68. *See also*
        community
        empowerment.
    knowledge of ADA rights, 56
Linton, Simi, 4

Marginalized groups,
and coalition building, 92-93
empowerment of, 92-93,111-112
inclusion in community coalitions,
92-93,111
research with, 4-5
Media involvement, 63,64,79
Minorities with disabilities, 55-56

National Council on Disability, *see*
Americans with Disabilities
Act
National Institute on Disability and
Rehabilitation Research
(NIDRR),
consumer involvement approach to
funding priorities, 17-19,
The Federal Register, 18
peer review panels, 19
National Institute of Health, 38
National Spinal Cord Injury
Association, 29
Needs assessment, 39-40,60,104,106.
See also Chronic fatigue
syndrome and Community
empowerment

Paralyzed Veterans of America,
27,29,30
Paraplegia News, 30
Participatory Action Research (PAR),
16-32
consumer-collaborators, 16,21
definition of, 16
implementation of, 21
interventions using,
See Action Letter Portfolio,
23-27
See Secondary conditions,
resources for preventing and
managing, 27-31
limitations of, 32
model of, 17-22
consumer-valued outcomes,

21-22,
ease of implementation, 21
quality of life, 21
social importance of, 21
external consumer influence,
17-19,
See also National Institute on
Disability and
Rehabilitation
Research, consumer
involvement
approach to funding
priorities
internal consumer influence,
Consumer Empowered Team,
19,31
utility of, 19
research process, 19-21
Consumer Concerns Report
Method, 20
and people with disabilities, 17
research using, 16-17
versus traditional research, 20
Participatory planning process, 102
People First language, 4
People with disabilities, *see also*
children with disabilities;
developmental disabilities;
physical disabilities; Chronic
Fatigue Syndrome;
Latino(a)s with disabilities;
Minorities with disabilities
abuse of, 3
communication barriers, 55-56
as co-researchers, 4,16-32
and discrimination, 55-56
employment of, 3,55,67
and equal access, 55
as home owners, 3
inclusion in community coalitions,
92-112
and independent living, 3,4
as a marginalized or minority
group, 3,4,92-93,111
prevalence of, 2
and research, 4,16,67

and transportation, 55
Physical disabilities, people with, 10
    and advocacy, 105
    research with, 20
PLAYS Recess program. *See also*
        Community Response Model
    capacity-building with community
        partners, 80-81
    data-based evaluation and
        participatory action research,
        82-83
    establishing a place in the system,
        78-79
    expansion to other schools, 86
    identification of needs and
        strengths, 77-78
    outcomes, 83-86
    positive visions, 81-82
    working relationship–a resource to
        the community, 79-80
Policymaking
    consumer input, 18-19
    setting priorities, 17-18
Positive visions, 8

Rappaport, Julian, 5,54,68
Rehabilitation Act (1973), 3,55
Researcher, as "learner," 16. *See also*
        Community Psychology
Research and Training Center in
    Independent Living
    (RTC/IL), 17,28,30,31
    Consumer Concerns Report
        Method, 20
Resource Team, 7-8
Riger, Stephanie, 111

Schools,
    identifying needs, 76-77
    interventions, 72-88, *see also* ACE
        Reading Program and
        PLAYS Recess Program
Secondary conditions,
    prevention and management of,
        28-30

resources for preventing and
    managing, 27-31,
    resource booklet, 28-29,31
    Second Thoughts, 29,31
Self-advocacy, 4
    advocacy action-planning guide, 64
    and the Americans with Disabilities
        Act, 22,54-68
    and empowerment, 56
    promoting self-advocacy skills, *see*
        Participatory Action
        research, Action Letter
        Portfolio
    and research, 4,67
    risks of self-advocacy, 64
Self-determination, 4,11
Self-help groups, 40,42-46
Socio-political definition of disability,
    39
Special education, 3,4,55,
    classification of children as
        children with disabilities,
        72,77
Spinal cord injury, 27,28
Spinal Cord Injury Education and
    Training Foundation, 27,28
Stakeholders, 73,74
Sustainability of interventions, 20,
    36,73

Technology, uses of, 80-81,87. *See
    also* Feedforward
Traditional research methods and
    evaluation, 12,20
Translations techniques, 61

Video futures, *see* Feedforward